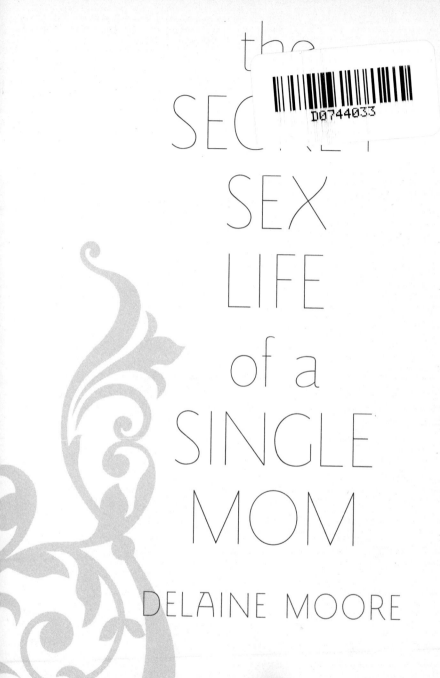

the SECRET SEX LIFE of a SINGLE MOM

DELAINE MOORE

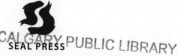

THE SECRET SEX LIFE OF A SINGLE MOM

Copyright © 2012 by Delaine Moore

Published by
Seal Press
A Member of the Perseus Books Group
1700 Fourth Street
Berkeley, California

Library of Congress Cataloging-in-Publication Data

Moore, Delaine, 1970-
  The secret sex life of a single mom / Delaine Moore.
      p. cm.
  ISBN 978-1-58005-386-0
  1. Single mothers—Social life and customs. 2. Single mothers—Sexual behavior. 3. Dating (Social customs) I. Title.
  HQ759.915.M63 2012
  306.874'32—dc23
                                    2011042224

Cover and interior design by Domini Dragoone
Printed in the United States of America
Distributed by Publishers Group West

To every Woman . . . and her Wild Woman

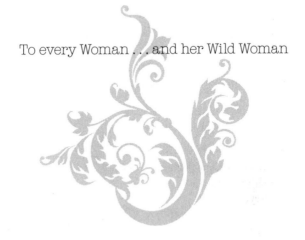

A Note from the Author

To preserve the anonymity of friends and lovers,
some names and identifying details have been changed.
However, the relationship mishaps and erotic
adventures are all mine and all true.

CONTENTS

Prologue 9

CHAPTER 1   Husbands and Lovers 13

CHAPTER 2   The Graham Bomb 33

CHAPTER 3   Online and Out of Line 39

CHAPTER 4   Friends in Need 49

CHAPTER 5   Afternoon Delight 59

CHAPTER 6   Stay-at-Home Mom Meets a Dom 71

CHAPTER 7   Red Light Means Go 81

CHAPTER 8   Chamber of Self-Doubt 101

CHAPTER 9   Sergeant Shane's Boot Camp 111

CHAPTER 10   Maneuvers and Touchdowns 119

CHAPTER 11   Operation Service Boy(s) 133

CHAPTER 12   Operation Double Satisfaction 151

CHAPTER 13   Hidden Desires and Hopefulness 159

CHAPTER 14   The Lioness Must Devour the Dik-Dik 167

CHAPTER 15   Ponytailed Mom vs. Audacious Online Diva 177

CHAPTER 16   Hotel Fantasy with a Service Male 183

CHAPTER 17   A Chameleon in Search of Home 191

CHAPTER 18   They Just Weren't That into Us 201

CHAPTER 19   Adventures in Wonderland 207

CHAPTER 20   The Dom and the Dragonfly 219

CHAPTER 21   Introductions to a New Year 235

CHAPTER 22   Boxed, Bound, and Delivered 251

CHAPTER 23   The Primary Shareholder of My Heart 271

Epilogue 281

EXTRACT

THE DUKE SAID IT WAS time for me to "stop talking" and "start walking." It was time to get out of his online classroom and take action in the real world. He wrote:

> By the time you're finished overanalyzing everything, not only will the cows have come home, they'll have had babies, and their babies will have had babies. If you want to find and exert your alpha-femaleness, you need to get out there.
>
> Think of it as having enlisted in a Sexuality Boot Camp, wherein I am your sergeant in command. Like a good little girl you will listen to your superior, and in turn, I'll make sure you keep your men in line—not to mention deliver good strong spankings when you're slacking off.
>
> What's that? Was that a "Yes Sir!"?

I laughed and thought, *How about "Bite me, sir."*

I leaned back in my chair, still smiling. *He sure does have a strange sense of humor.* But for whatever reason, *I liked it.* I liked that he caught me off guard, and I liked that he made me lighten up around the realm of dating and sex.

Shane's proposition appealed to me, despite the fact it was totally unconventional. Not taking every date seriously seemed a pretty sensible thing for me to do right now, because it liberated me to have fun and explore. Maybe my need to "seek and replace" wasn't as urgent as I once thought. Surely it wouldn't hurt to delay it a month or two . . .

I hit the reply button, smirking and shaking my head. *Yes, I think I'll play along with "Sergeant Shane."* Temporarily, anyway. Or unless Mr. Right comes along . . .

PROLOGUE

IF YOU LOOKED AT MY life from the outside, you would never assume I was any different than most middle-class suburban women my age—a self-sacrificing wife and mother.

In my case, I have three children: two boys and one girl, who are six, five, and three. And I drive a wickedly practical minivan: a blue Honda filled with crumbs and stray toy parts.

Yes, I am rarely alone in it. And yes, I've driven in my pajamas (thank God for long coats).

Almost seven years ago, I willingly abandoned my just-taking-off career as a cognitive therapist to pursue a vocation as a stay-at-home mom and housewife. I've worked hard, and I'm proud of the job I've done raising my kids almost single-handedly. Their father, a land developer, was out of town 80 percent of the time.

No, it was never my big dream growing up to be a homemaker. If anything, I thought I'd be light years ahead of my mom's generation, finding complete fulfillment in some creative, dynamic career.

But when Robert and my babies came along, I readily changed all my goals and plans; I fell hard in love with the family dream.

Motherhood shook and rocked me to the core, in ways I was

totally unprepared for. I suddenly understood the true meaning of unconditional love: not only was it a feeling, it was a verb that required twenty-four-hour attention. In my limited spare time, when I wasn't catering to my kids or my husband, I read parenting books, organized mom groups, researched educational programs; there was *always* more to do and learn, and I eagerly applied myself. Motherhood filled me with a purpose—a higher purpose—for life wasn't just about me anymore . . . my world, my consciousness, had expanded a hundredfold.

That's not to say I found my job *easy*—it also drove me a little nuts—sometimes several times a day. There's nothing like getting everyone packed up in snowsuits and strapped into the van (finally!), only to have someone pee their pants. Or to exit a shopping mall with three crying, screaming kids in tow: one refusing to walk, one in a football hold, and one in a stroller.

But I chose to focus on the blessings and rewards of my toils; I knew this stage of my life wouldn't be forever, that there were many wonderful lessons in it for me—such as developing the virtue of patience and learning to live in the now. I knew that, overall, motherhood was molding me into a better woman.

There were only two things I consistently did for *myself* during this time: maintain close relationships with my circle of girlfriends (even if it was primarily by phone), and work out at the gym (which had great childcare). Not only did exercise briefly relieve me from mommy duty, it resurrected my pelvic floor *and* kept me relatively toned everywhere else.

I sure am glad I prioritized those two things now . . .

You see, I was hurled into singlehood again. Only this time with three kids and big responsibilities in tow. Life as I'd known it was gone—flattened by the tornado of betrayal.

But out of this wreckage, I constructed a new life of liberation—one built on the foundation of my profound, dare I say unconventional, sexual awakening. But I kept my provocative dating and sex life deliberately secret to avoid becoming headline news among other mothers on the school playground. After all, thirty-something suburban moms did *not* go to sex clubs or meet young men for afternoon trysts. Or did they . . . ?

From online dating to domination and submission, I barely left a stone unturned in my quest to explore the boundaries not only of my sexuality but of myself. And in so doing, I experienced more than just wild adventures—I excavated my authentic and fiery self. The Delaine who had once defined herself as mother and wife rediscovered Delaine the Woman, without sacrificing motherhood.

It all began with a phone call in the night . . .

CHAPTER 1

HUSBANDS
AND LOVERS

It was the night before Halloween. I was half-asleep, half-awake, nursing my six-month-old daughter, Jessa, when the phone rang. I raced to answer it, Jessa still attached to my breast.

"Is Robert there?" asked an unfamiliar voice. It was a woman, her speech slurred from drinking.

"No, he's not, he's away at work," I said automatically. I wiped a long strand of hair out of my eyes and glanced at the clock: 3:25 AM. "Who *is* this?"

Husky giggles. "Just a friend."

"Pardon? *Just a* friend?" My brain was fully alert now.

"I'm sorry, *who* are you again?"

Click.

I held the receiver out from my ear and stared at it. My arms and fingers suddenly felt numb. *What the hell just happened? Who the hell was she?!* I laid my daughter down in her crib and called the number back, heart racing, my bloodstream prickling with ice.

"Chubbie's Bar and Grill," said a lively male voice, loud over the din of background music.

Gripping the phone tighter, I put on my best casual/happy voice. "Hi, I just received a call from a woman at this number. She was asking for my husband, Robert Williams. Can I speak with her please?"

"Oh . . . ummm . . . that was Natasha." Muffled sounds followed. He had covered the mouthpiece, but I could still hear him talking to someone in the background: "Man . . . that was a really stupid move . . . "

"Hello? Hey . . . " I called.

"Yeah, hi. Sorry. Listen . . . " he began to say, but I cut him off.

"Do *you* know my husband?"

More muffled sounds.

Again, more forcefully: "Do you know my husband, *Robert Williams?*"

His answer was immediate.

"Yes."

"Is there something going on between her and my husband?" I felt my fear rising, mixed with panic, and the telltale flood of emotion welling up behind both. I took a deep breath, trying desperately to calm myself.

Silence.

"Please," I implored, softening. "Please tell me. I am his wife, we have *three children*. Is there something going on?" But he didn't need to tell me. Instinct told me my answer. My hope was that the Chubbie's man would prove me wrong.

Silence.

"Please," I begged. "Are you a dad?"

Exhale. "Yes."

"Then *please*, PLEASE, tell me. We have a newborn baby, a two-year-old, and *(choke)* a three-year-old."

Finally: "You should look into it."

I ran to the bathroom and threw up.

In a daze, I stumbled back to the phone and called Robert, who was at his new job site, a six hour's drive west.

"Hello," he answered groggy with sleep.

"So . . . your girlfriend just called," I said matter-of-factly. My whole body trembled and my heart raced. The moment felt surreal, like I was acting out a movie script, because how could I be asking my Robert about his *girlfriend?* He was my husband. My *love.* I swallowed back a sob as I waited for his response.

"What? What do you mean?"

But I didn't answer. He'd heard me. He knew what I meant. I just stared at the wall in front of me, my eyes locked on a red crayon mark I hadn't scrubbed off.

"Delaine, answer me . . . DELAINE . . . Oh fuck . . ." He sounded panicked, but I didn't care—or feel anything. "I'm coming home right now, Delaine, okay? I'm getting in my truck *right now* and coming home," he said, as if trying to reassure me.

Later that day when I saw his truck pull into the driveway, I was waiting at the door: I waved goodbye to the kids and the sitter, got in the front seat without looking at him, and he drove for what felt like hours, up a twisting road, both of us quiet. Occasionally, I'd look over at him, at his familiar profile, his rugged handsome jawline, and I'd feel a fresh punch to my gut, my eyes quickly pooling with tears. *Oh Robert,* I wanted to sob, *how could you do this to us?* But I couldn't give in to emotion; I didn't want my weakness to get in the way of knowing everything. The road gave out finally on an empty construction lot high atop a hill overlooking the city. He turned off the engine, and the truck was flooded with silence.

He shifted in the leather seat, and looked at me with a soft expression, loving, remorseful even. I looked out the window, waiting . . . bracing myself for what was to come.

"Nothing happened Delaine," he pleaded softly. "I swear to God nothing happened. She's just a friend, and she means absolutely nothing to me. If you don't want me to see her again, I won't."

I turned and looked at him, holding his gaze. He looked away, out the front window, then down at his hands. *"Nothing* happened?" I asked beseechingly, tissues knotted in my hands. "You didn't even kiss her?"

He didn't speak immediately. Eyes out the window. Long exhale. Finally: "Yes. I'll be honest. I did kiss her. But only once." He looked at me, his face earnest. "I swear to God, Delaine. Just *once.*"

Fresh tears streamed down my face; visions of Robert amorously entwined with another woman.

But I believed him—it was just a kiss. It was but one small, insignificant mistake . . .

"YOU KNOW THAT's bullshit, right?" retorted my best friend, Hali, when I relayed Robert's story to her the next day.

"Huh?" I sat on the couch, my arms moving to wrap around my knees. "What do you mean?"

Hali's face softened, and she reached for my hand. "Delaine," she said gently. "Look . . . I know you want to believe him. And it's wonderful that you want to give him the benefit of the doubt. But do you *really* think full-grown men stop at a kiss? If he was ten or twelve years old, maybe. But a horny adult male who knows how good sex feels? Hon, he's lying."

No. *No.* My world was crashing to the ground in slow motion. I needed answers. I needed the truth, but I knew I wouldn't get it from him; I had to talk to *her.*

WE SAT ACROSS from each other at Chubbie's Bar and Grill, where she worked as a bar manager. I listened quietly, determined not to cry, while she nervously, yet openly, answered my questions. Thoughts distracted me: Robert kissing her full lips, Robert running his hands through her long dark hair, the two of them giggling and pillow-talking in the afterglow of sex. *Robert knows every inch of this woman's body*, I thought, glancing down at her full breasts and trim waistline, untouched by pregnancy. I felt plain and matronly in my cords and T-shirt.

Finally, with my eyes across the room, I asked the one question that haunted me most: "Did he ever say he loved you?"

She inhaled deeply and flicked her cigarette. Finally: "No. But we spent a lot of time together. We were really good friends, and we cared *a lot* about each other." She was nodding her head, staring down at the table. When she finally looked up into my eyes, I saw straight into her pain: *She'd* fallen in love with *him*. This young, smart, and obviously beautiful woman before me had secretly believed he would choose her over us.

I never spoke with her again.

IN RETROSPECT, I saw there had been signs. The new sex maneuvers he tried, which I assumed he'd read about in a magazine. Going to the tanning booth in winter. And ah yes . . . all those extra showers, which I'd assumed were out of consideration for me. Perhaps someone swifter, brighter, or not so insanely busy would've pounced on these clues right away. But I trusted him. Completely. I simply didn't think he was the kind of man who would ever cheat.

Sure, I knew Robert and I had some problems in our marriage. Who doesn't when they have a young family? I thought that Robert and I were simply going through a life phase that required a lot more energy and sacrifice, where the "us" in the equation took a backseat to the more pressing needs of newborns and toddlers. In my mind, we'd shared and built so much together— good stuff, important stuff, too meaningful to ever put at risk: a home, three precious children, a community of friends, and a partnership which was built on strong family values. Granted, we argued on occasion, he could be unkind and demanding, unyielding and insensitive. But at the time, I overlooked these failings for the greater good of our family unit. Never once did I think he might be cheating on me.

I resolved I'd forgive him. Somehow, even though my soul was battered, I forced myself to try and understand Robert's unhappiness, the reasons why he had made these choices. I believed my family's future was contingent upon my ability to forgive. So I determined I would.

Over the next year, we took all the right steps to slowly rebuild: counseling, dating each other more often, exploring new common hobbies. He communicated more, drank and swore less. He participated in family time and turned off his cell phone. He tried to be present, to make amends. And I loved him for trying. I felt compassion for him, like a mother might feel for a child who's made a bad choice. But the one thing I couldn't do was bring myself to have sex with him, because under the surface, everything had changed.

BEFORE THE AFFAIR, Robert and I had had regular sex—that is, about three or four times a week when he wasn't traveling. But I carried what I felt was a terrible secret: Just the thought of Robert's sexual touch made me inwardly cringe. No matter what I tried, my body seemed to rebuff him. I tried watching porn and masturbating beforehand. I even tried alcohol. Still . . . baseline. I'd fill my heart with appreciation for him; I'd admire his tall, muscular body as he stepped out of the shower, glistening and wet. Still nothing.

The truth was that my body started rejecting Robert as far back as my first pregnancy. Robert would come home after working out of town for weeks, horny as a raging bull, and I would be tired, throwing up from morning sickness, feeling no desire whatsoever. But I quickly discovered that saying no to sex meant emotional retaliation: "What happened to the girl who liked to do it three times a day?" he snarled at me once. "What's wrong with you?"

"*All* couples at the start of a relationship have loads of sex Robert," I said beseechingly. "It's normal for it to tone down over time."

"Well it's not normal to me!" he spat angrily. "It's false representation. Christ, it really is true: As soon as you're married and the woman has you by the balls, she cuts off sex."

His comments stung. They were cruel and selfish, but I also felt guilty for not satisfying him. My bruised emotions notwithstanding, the loyal do-gooder wife in me wondered if he was somehow right. By marrying me, he had forsaken all other women under the faith that I would adequately meet his sexual needs. Yes, I had a responsibility to fulfill that obligation, but was my sexual disinterest par for the course in marriage, especially after having kids—or was it just me?

Confused, I asked Hali what her and her husband, Paul's, sex life was like. They'd been married ten years at the time, so the honeymoon phase was certainly over. I figured her reality would be pretty representative of mine.

When I asked her, at first she laughed. We were sitting in my bright cluttered kitchen, our toddlers running rampant through the house. As always, she looked fresh and eye-catchingly pretty, her naturally blonde pixie cut flattering her delicate features and blue eyes. But underneath her ultrafeminine exterior lay a kind but no-bullshit woman, one who had an opinion and was more than ready to offer it up. When we'd first met ten years earlier, neither one of us much liked the other: She thought me a rather free-spirited "hippie," and I found her uncomfortably frank, which, at the time, made her seem harsh around the edges. But we openly laughed about that now. I think our differences helped cement our friendship because we saw something in each other that we needed in ourselves.

"No, I'm serious, Hali," I said, laughing too.

"Okay, okay, D," she said, rolling her eyes. "Let's see, I'd say it's predictable, but okay. Nothing to write home about. I get into it once I get going." She paused, tilted her head. "Actually, whenever I have a great orgasm I think, 'why don't we do this more often?' But my problem is getting to the point where I *want* to get going: I'm tired, I feel fat, he has bad breathe, whatever. Suddenly, I'll realize we haven't had sex in a month."

"But what about when he approaches you and you're not in the mood? Do you feel guilty if you say no?" I picked at a bowl of grapes, which the kids had already attacked. The few stragglers were overripe. I popped them in my mouth absentmindedly as I listened to Hali's answer.

"Not really. I mean, if he needs it that bad he can go do his thing in the bathroom," she said dryly.

I laughed so hard, I nearly shot grape skin out my nose.

"But is that fair?" I pressed further. "I mean, aren't we supposed to make the extra effort out of respect to our husbands? Chances are we're not always going to be in the mood at the same time."

"I see what you mean," she replied, taking a moment to think. "Actually . . . yeah, I sometimes do have sex more for him than me. But like I said, once we get going, I usually get into it."

I FOUND SOLACE in knowing other people's sex lives weren't perfect either. *Marriage will always present us with one challenge or another,* I thought, with resignation. I just needed to hang tough, focus on my blessings, and stay true to the course.

And that's when I made a dangerous choice: To keep the peace between Robert and me, I would simply give in. Yield. Detach. Pretend . . .

Oh, he's looking at your face—smile! Make your eyes look alive.

Offer him a blowjob, then at least you can plan your day or week in the interim.

Stare at that little crack again in the ceiling. Imagine floating up there . . .

And so on.

Once I started pretending, my sex drive never came back. Even though we went on to have two more children, and even though I believed I loved Robert, I simply tolerated having sex with him.

After his affair, as we worked with a counselor, I silently, anxiously, hoped that my sexual passion would reignite, that all this would bring us closer together and be the catalyst to renewed passion. Two months passed; nothing. Then three . . . four . . . five. Still, I felt absolutely no desire. But I knew I couldn't expect him to wait forever. *He's trying so hard to be a better husband and dad. He deserves to have sex again,* I reasoned. *The problem really is mine.*

So one night, I decided it was time. I mustered my courage, carefully dressed up in something lacy and seductive, and served myself to him like a plate of chicken.

He loved it. I felt nothing.

As we moved toward the one year mark of his affair, I resigned myself to thinking I would never enjoy sex again. For the rest of my life, it would be something to "get over with." I told myself I didn't *need* to enjoy sex. It was overrated and there were other, more important things, like keeping my family together. In fact, I imagined many of my foremothers had felt the same way. In my mind's eye, I'd see a farm wife falling exhausted into bed after an eighteen-hour day of chores and caring for her ten kids . . . only to be awoken, yet again, by her husband's calloused fingers under her bed dress. This was all just a part of marriage. A part of life. Besides, look how happy having sex made *him*—I'd literally find him whistling around the house, more than willing to do chores. And he was kinder, less harsh. Giving him my body seemed like such a small price to pay.

AROUND THIS TIME, a terrible pain in my hip appeared out of nowhere. It was interfering with my sleep and growing worse by the week. Thus, almost one year after Robert's affair, I began twice-weekly treatments with a highly reputed acupuncturist named Graham, a tall, lean, Zen-looking man with unkempt dark hair and gentle eyes. From the moment I met him in the waiting room, I felt at ease by his warm smile and calm presence.

One day, as he worked on my hip in a session, I suddenly found myself crying. "My God, this is so embarrassing," I apologized, as he quickly offered me a tissue. "Watching the leaves fall, Halloween just around the corner—they remind me of painful events from last year."

Graham rolled his stool close to me and sat down, like he was fully prepared to listen to what I had to say. I could feel his presence, his attention, his kind brown eyes upon me. No pressure . . . no conditions. Just his powerfully gentle care.

The words poured from my mouth like blood out of a fresh wound. I told him of Robert's betrayal, every detail. And as I told my story to Graham—who, despite all logic, felt like a trusted longtime friend—I wept like a grief-stricken child.

A dozen tissues later, I finally composed myself. "I'm really sorry to make such a scene," I said self-consciously. "I don't understand why this had to come out today, or here in your office."

Graham looked upward for a moment, as if gathering his words from some otherworldly source. "The body never lies, Delaine," he said, his soft baritone voice full of compassion. "Our bodies know and feel our truth, even when our minds aren't there yet. You suffered tremendously, and your pain has manifested in your body. It needed to come out. Today's session just triggered it."

That night as I lay in bed, my body felt exhausted, yet lighter. It was as if I'd released something, and in its place was a serene weariness.

But then Robert came into the bedroom.

Immediately, I tensed from head to toe. I lay still, pretending to sleep. He crawled into bed and rolled over on to his side. I listened to his breathing, lying motionless, frozen, until I could tell he was asleep.

As I stared at the ceiling, Graham's words came back to me: *"The body never lies . . ."*

OVER THE NEXT few months of treatment with Graham, my body began telling me something *else*: I was intensely attracted to him. No, it wasn't just because of his lean runner's body and dark, chiseled features; I swear I hardly even noticed his good looks when we first met. My attraction grew slowly, innocently, out of the conversations we shared. His mind, his energy, his sensitivity crept into known and unknown places within me . . . and filled them with light. He never crossed any professional lines, but sometimes, sometimes . . . during breaks in our conversations, he'd look down at me, and our eyes would meet and hold. I could swear I saw equal desire reflected back in his.

I tried to fight my feelings. I minimized them, denied them, even berated myself for them. But he was so different from Robert—a complete and total opposite. Side by side, they were like New Age Healer and an Old School Brute. Graham was expressive and attentive; he showed his strength through acts and words of gentleness. Robert, on the other hand, was crass and domineering, more apt to down a bottle of whisky or pull a wheelie on his motorcycle to prove his manhood. Mentally, I could connect with Graham with such ease; I marveled at how a thirty-minute session could pass so quickly, especially when someone was poking me with needles. And the fact that he, too, was adrift in a failing marriage with an emotionally distant wife, clinging to the hope that it might someday turn a corner for the sake of his three kids, was yet one more thing we had in common.

I struggled with my feelings constantly, torn between fantasy and reality, truth and deceit, right and wrong. I knew I should stop seeing him as my therapist and firmly walk away, but I simply couldn't fight it; I didn't *want* to fight it. And in a flash, I understood the roots of Robert's indiscretion.

We arranged our first rendezvous at a hotel close by. I was drunk on two glasses of wine when he arrived, and he looked around so conspicuously, that I was sure the front desk clerk must have known. We knew we were crossing a formidable moral line, one that carried a dangerous price tag if we were caught. Still, we proceeded. We had no future expectations of one another, no promises, only the mutual need to be together this one time.

Ah, but to finally be alone together—to finally allow the flesh to express the connection that had grown between us for months. We stood before one another kissing long and tenderly. God how I'd ached for this. How I'd longed to feel his arms around me, his lean chest pressing against mine.

Yet he was trembling; his entire six-foot-three frame was visibly shaking. "I'm sorry," he offered softy, his dark eyes beseeching mine. "I want to do this, I really want you, Delaine. It's just *such* a big step."

"Shhh, it's okay," I replied, looking up at him. "I'm really nervous too . . ." And with our admissions came laughter: "Boy, aren't we the most pathetic pair of cheaters," he grinned. And with laughter, the pressure seemingly disappeared; for when he reached down to kiss me again, there was no more shaking, only the undeniable presence of his passion.

And I allowed him to take the lead. I allowed him to bring me across that line with him. Because I wanted him; my body wanted him.

One night would never be enough.

MY SEX DRIVE exploded back like a neutron hitting plutonium. *Who* is *this woman?* I laughed at myself. My body craved sex so intensely and frequently it baffled me. Just the mere thought of Graham filled me with longing, an ache that surged deep inside my pelvis and stretched up to my heart.

Not only was I enjoying sex again, all the creative energies associated with my sex chakra were streaming throughout my being: Vibrancy! Effervescence! Passion! I couldn't even remember the last time I'd felt such things! I mean, it wasn't that my life as Robert's wife didn't make me feel "happy." It just felt more along the lines of . . . contentedness. Not bad, not good. Just "content." Or was it complacency?

However I labeled it, I believed my feelings were par for the marriage course—that as the banality of life settled in, as I assumed it did in most marriages, the arc of passion and magic fell away. This was all part of the natural order of things. I'd developed such beliefs in order to normalize what I was experiencing—or maybe endure it, I don't know. But I thought my ultimate job, my marital duty, was to appreciate what I *did* have, put honor and society's morality code above all else, and trust that over time mine and my husband's virtuous behavior would translate into "happily ever after." I bought the marriage sacrament hook, line, and sinker. It didn't occur to me that it could be any different.

But now, my passion was back. My dull, mediocre existence was dancing in color, a full-blown sensory experience painted with pleasure and beauty. And that's when my inspired energy met opportunity: Out of the blue, I decided to create my own Internet business. "Pregnant Soul," in how I dreamed it, would be unlike any other pregnancy site: it would take the emphasis off the physical journey of pregnancy and focus on nurturing the mother in the making.

My new business venture meant the world to me—not just for the creative outlet it provided, but for the new self-image it was birthing. I'd been out of the workforce for seven years, and my self-confidence was shaky at best. Maybe there was a smart, dynamic business woman lurking beneath my Supermom attire. My creative energies, now channeled into a goal, fuelled me with a new purpose in life.

As months slowly folded into a year, there came the day when I knew I was in love with Graham. I was peacefully snuggled up on his chest after having made love. The room was completely silent beside the sound of his heartbeat. Then he spoke.

"You are like a beautiful butterfly, Delaine," he said softly. "One that was trapped in her cocoon for a very long time . . ." He was stroking my hair as we talked, and I felt such tenderness, something I hadn't ever truly felt with Robert. "I've watched you transform these past months we've been together. . . I've watched you grow these exquisite, colorful wings. All you needed was a bit more time and someone to *really* love you."

My throat closed. I pressed my face deeper into his chest, as my heart absorbed the beauty of his words. Gently, he continued: "*Now* the question is: *Does she believe she can fly?* She can, you know. She just needs to trust and believe . . . in *herself*."

He lifted my face to his and kissed me.

In that brief moment, I realized I never wanted to be apart from this man; that we connected—mind, body, and soul—in a way Robert and I never had and never would. This was not some foolhardy, childish romance, I told myself. Nor was it just a sexually driven affair. To me, it was the real thing—kindred love; yin and yang, on all levels. And I believed Graham felt the same.

But of course, things couldn't go on as they were forever. The bottom line was that Graham and I were still married to other people. I was doing what Robert had done, even though I justified it by love. We were committing adultery, and choices inevitably had to be made. But first I needed to stop running. I needed to face off with two scary questions that had chased me for years; questions that were being posed by a most mistrusted source: my body. *Why do you dislike having sex with your husband, Delaine? And could it ever change for the better?*

I'd always tried to blame our sexual disconnection on me—*my* hormones, my feeling fat, my being pregnant, my being selfish. But now my body was standing firm and calling bullshit.

Flashback: *I am on my knees in front of the toilet bowl, three months pregnant with our first child. I have just thrown up for the sixth time that day. Suddenly, movement at the bathroom door catches my eye.*

He is standing there.

Naked.

Touching himself.

"Are you done yet?" he asks impatiently. "C'mon baby—let's get it on!"

My stomach lurches. Tears fill my eyes. "I'll be there in a second," I say, looking down. I pull myself up off the floor, brush my teeth, and proceed to our bedroom to fulfill my "wifely duty."

My body boiled with rage at the memory. How dare he have demanded sex when I was sick as a dog from carrying his child? Then my anger surged back at me*: Why didn't you just damn well say no? You enabled it, Delaine! Not just once but over and over and over again!*

Flashback: *We'd just finished having sex and I am lying in bed, watching him dress. An "aha" question suddenly hits me: "Robert," I ask, sitting up. "Do you enjoy having so much sex because it makes you feel close to me?"*

He looks at me funny, then continues putting on his socks.

"I'm serious," I say, leaning in. "Have you ever wondered if it's through sex that you feel most connected to me? Maybe it's the primary way you show love?"

He pauses for a moment, then laughs: "Nah. I just need to get off."

There it was. In his own words: "I just need to get off." But did I hear him? Did I listen? No. Instead I chose to psychoanalyze him, me, us: "It's a Mars/Venus thing" or "It's just a stage in marriage" or "It's a case of mismatched sex drives." How about, "Your husband doesn't respect you, Delaine . . . and neither do you."

I'd always tried to have a positive outlook and focus on the good things about Robert and our relationship beyond the bedroom. But they didn't erase his Dark Side—a side I'd chosen to make excuses for in the name of love, and family.

He's younger than me and more immature. He'll eventually grow up . . .

He doesn't know how to communicate because no one in his family can . . .

He doesn't really mean it when he says those things . . .

I maintained that his criticisms never hurt me, even though virtually nothing was off-limits to his attacks: my cooking, my friends, my family, my competence, my parenting skills, my appearance. *I can take it,* I would tell myself. *I'm just more self-aware than he is, but he'll get there.*

Of course, I was lying to myself. Over time, the negative bombardment had silently chipped away at my soul *and* my body—those restless dreams, the unexplained muscle pains, the heaviness in my chest, and yes, the absence of sexual desire. Underneath my skin I felt squashed. Belittled. Unheard. At some point or another, I'd started convincing myself I was happy, instead of facing the truth: I was living in denial and subsisting off of self-told lies.

The body never lies. Such poignancy in those words now. My sexual self had literally closed to Robert as a means of self-protection. My body had learned long ago what my mind and heart had been unprepared to acknowledge: My marriage was severely broken. And Robert's infidelity had yielded the final blow.

Even though I had forgiven him, even though I could still

laugh and carry on a conversation with him, that was as far as I could extend it. My body had had *enough*. I knew I would never feel special with him, a feeling I wanted, needed, and deserved. Moreover, I knew such a feeling was possible because I believed in soul mates, and the universe had reunited me with Graham.

"I TOLD ROBERT I want a divorce," I said to Graham the day after it happened. It was a cold December day and we'd snuck away to share tea at a coffee shop.

"You *did*?" He was surprised.

"I did. It was hard. And he was very sad. But I know it's the right decision."

"Wow. Good for you, Delaine. That's such a big step to take. You're a very courageous woman." He looked away. "Let's hope your separation goes better than mine." Graham was already deep in the throes of his, and it had turned nasty because of money matters.

"Can I come over to your new condo tonight? I still haven't seen it since you moved out."

"Actually, I've been thinking . . ." He took a deep breath. "I think you and I need to take some time apart. Not forever, just for now. Things are becoming so complicated at home. And if Maria catches wind of us, she will make my life even more of a living hell."

His words caught me off guard.

"Delaine," he said, gathering my hands in his own. "You know I love you. But because of that, I don't want you to hear about all the ugliness going on between me and Maria. I don't want it to taint us."

I was nodding because his words made sense, but they still hurt. I had to absorb them.

Graham continued, his jaw set: "This is such a major life transition—for both of us. And I need to be able to stand on my own two feet and work things out for myself, as do you. The easy thing to do is to run for shelter in a lover's arms where it all feels good. But against such an ugly backdrop? It might ruin us before we have a real chance to be together."

"So you don't want any physical contact either?" I asked. *Yearning.*

"I think it's best if we don't, Delaine. I want to honey, God, I *want* to. But it's dangerous. And at this stage of things, we need to be so careful."

I was upset. But at the time, I believed in his devotion, so I saw the wisdom in his words. We needed to be strong and close these chapters of our lives on our own.

Over the next four months our communication was very limited—only a couple of phone calls per month and a few coffee dates with whispered I love you's. I coped by filling my daydreams and nights with memories and hope-filled visions of our future. I also made certain there was room in my heart to welcome and love his three children as my own.

I focused my attention on dismantling my own marriage. The whole separation process felt surreal, like a drawn-out death. It's a time when hostility and anger can flare at the drop of a hat, fear takes over, and anxiety prevails. To curtail my own, I avoided talking to people who had already gone through a messy divorce. I alone had chosen to arrive at this major crossroads in my life. And despite my many fears, I trusted in myself to find my own way.

Sometimes though, my grief at what was transpiring completely overwhelmed me. I had to give in to it and find a quiet time and place to release it. I looked around me to the rhythms of nature, knowing that every moment, the cycle of birth, death, and renewal was ongoing; and I drew comfort from it. I knew that our relationship was not so much ending as transforming. From the ashes of our marriage, our new roles as coparents, and hopefully friends, would emerge.

I finally knew which direction my life was heading; I'd made a choice. At some not-too-far juncture, I foresaw reuniting with Graham and the merging of our families. I sent Graham my prayers and loving thoughts, and I patiently awaited his freedom.

CHAPTER 2

THE GRAHAM BOMB

OF ALL THE MOTHERS I'D met at my sons' school that year, Sara was the only one I'd become close enough with to call a real friend.

It was over lunch with her one day in March that I confided that Robert and I had separated. I was selective about who I told at that point, mostly because I was afraid of being judged and seen as a failure; I couldn't handle that extra burden. I needed time and space to process my grief. Sometimes it completely overwhelmed me, and I'd be flooded with all the good memories of us as a family—the teary look on Robert's face as he held our first child, family snuggles in our bed, all of us linked hand-in-hand as we walked, Robert looking at me with love in his eyes—my younger self loving him with such abandon. But harder still was mourning the death of the "dream," to have believed and worked so hard and for so long at something, only to be letting it go.

As I sat across from Sara that day over lunch, briefly discussing my separation from Robert, I impulsively decided to tell her I'd met someone else—"a most captivating man named Graham." I described him to her only briefly, when she suddenly asked, "Does he run?"

"Yes!" I replied, surprised. "Oh my god, do you *know* him?" I felt a little self-conscious suddenly, like she was seeing deeper into my life than I intended. But I was also oddly excited, because a part of me was bursting to tell the world about my secret true love.

"Well, yes, but not well. I went running with him and a mutual friend once. Whew, he is one *fast* runner, talk about being in a great shape. I couldn't keep up! We both laughed, marveling over what a small "big city" it was.

A few weeks later, I was hurrying to pick up my son at school and passed Sarah in the hall. "Delaine!" she called out. "There's something I need to tell you. Come talk to me after you get your son."

Something in her voice stopped me in my tracks. I hurried back to her. "No. It's okay, I have a quick sec. Kalob's teacher always stays late. What is it?"

"It's about Graham," she said, looking pained.

My heart jumped, and I felt a sudden wash of dread.

"There's no easy way to tell you this so I'm just going to say it; I think you need to know. Graham has been having an affair with another woman for the past nine months. But it's more than that," she added quickly, as I opened my mouth to speak. "She's having his baby in three weeks."

"*What?*" I said, completely taken aback. I was shaking my head no, my brain trying to connect nonexistent dots. Wait. This must be some weird, freaky misunderstanding. *Of course!* She had the wrong man.

"No, that's not possible," I laughed. "You must know another Graham. Oh my god, you totally scared me," I said, pressing my hand against my heart. "No, my Graham already has kids—three of them—and he specializes in acupressure, over in Sunnydale."

Sara was nodding. *Why is she nodding,* I thought, confused. "Yes. That's him, Delaine. That's Graham. I know him. The girl he got pregnant is also my friend. The one we went running with."

Time stood still. I couldn't breathe. It wasn't possible. This was *preposterous.* We talked a bit more . . . a few more details she couldn't have known, like his children's names. Everything she said was true. How could she know? *Oh my God, oh my god, please don't make it true!* My body was shaking and my stomach heaved upward, pressing my heart, my soul, my future against the back of my throat. I was sure I would vomit and never stop. *My son! I have to pick up my son* . . . yes, there he is, smile at him, hold his hand, walk home . . . Fuck me, fuck, fuck, *fuck.* RUN! sobbed my body and my head. Fucking *run* . . .

But there was nowhere to run, and no one to run to. And thus, as my son and I made our way home, past rows of minivan moms shoveling backpacks and kids into cars, I felt my heart explode in my chest.

I settled the kids with the baby sitter as quickly as possible then retreated to the bathroom and locked the door. There, on the shower mat, I curled against the despair and let my body do its best to purge itself of pain. Then, a single unrelenting thought possessed me: *I have to confront him.* Absolutely nothing else mattered besides that thought. I stepped into the shower, washing the film of tears off my face, and went through the motions of making myself look pretty. I got in my minivan, feeling oddly tethered, and drove to his work.

When I saw his truck in the parking lot, a fresh wave of anguish enveloped me: *How many times had I ridden beside him in that truck, holding his hand?* I wondered. I parked beside it. And waited.

I saw him before he saw me, his tall frame filling up the glass door as he exited.

I waited until he'd opened the door to his truck before I marched up to him on legs that were void of sensation. "You owe me an explanation."

He smiled brightly—*very* surprised. "What're you doing here?" he said, looking confused. "And what are you talking about?" He was shaking his head, apparently clueless.

"You owe me an explanation. About *Melissa.*"

In the flash of a second, his face turned grey and his demeanor stiffened. "Get in," he ordered. "We can't do this here." He drove to the furthest side of the lot and parked.

At first he denied it. Then he minimized it and left out important facts. But I knew to dig deeper, to hunt for lies—visions of Robert's lame-assed confession loomed in my mind; kind of sick it had unfolded in his truck, too. Eventually, I had Graham confirm almost everything Sara had told me.

Finally, a moment of pause, no tears. As we sat there, the sky dark around us, rain started pouring down on the windshield. I looked down at my hands and my knotted up tissues. The tears recommenced flowing, heavily but silently.

I turned and looked at him, my voice raw with hurt. "How *could* you? How could you do this to me? All I've ever done is love you and show you how much I love you. After all that you know about me, after knowing I just went through this with Robert, how *could* you?"

More than anything, I needed an answer. Let him tell me something self-analytical, something comforting, something insightful and rational.

But he just sat there, his jaw stiff, staring out the window. Rain poured down.

"You've been having sex with another woman and she's about to have your *baby.* You've deliberately kept my life on hold. You should have told me, you should have *set me free.* Why didn't you? *Why?*"

His face was a torment of emotions, but he remained silent.

"Answer me!" I half yelled, half choked.

"I didn't know how to tell you!" he blurted. "I didn't know how because I have no balls, okay? *I have no balls.* I'm sorry, Delaine. I swear I *do* love you. I'm so sorry. I never meant to hurt you."

And that was it. That was all he could come up with. This man, whom I thought was the greatest, wisest, most magnificent man I'd ever met, apparently *loved* me . . . but *had no balls*.

And thus it was that April 2 became my personal D-Day, as yet *another* man not only chopped up my heart, but tossed me, wrecked, into a singlehood I'd never even considered. I felt dead; thirty-seven and dead, with three young kids, and a divorce underway.

I WENT THROUGH the motions of my day-to-day life. I had to force myself to eat. It hurt to smile. It hurt to get out of bed. It hurt to have no interest in my kids, who had been the center of my heart and existence for so long. Mommy was a shell of a woman. Could they tell?

I felt guilty for not being able to put them first, *before* me and my pain, like a good mother should. I felt guilty for not wanting to go into their imaginary worlds to play and for leaving them with my baby sitter more often so I could simply survive another day. But my guilt just blended with my numbness. My mind, body, and soul were empty.

So I reached for cigarettes to comfort me. Who cares if I'd quit for seven years? I didn't want to breathe deeply or feel any deeper inside me than I already was.

I knew that loving someone purely and abundantly was nothing to be ashamed of. But my God, all my "knowing" wasn't helping me pull myself back together. I felt like fragments of my being were sticking out of me in all the wrong places. I had totally fallen out of alignment, and I didn't know how to put Delaine back together again. Where was all that higher understanding and faith I had worked so hard to accumulate over my life? *Now* was the time for me to be drawing it forth and leaning on it. Where'd it go?

But I didn't have the energy to quiet my mind and meditate. I didn't have the focus or interest in reading any self-help books.

I couldn't look to nature or the radiant faces of my children to stay present in the moment; I couldn't find peace in a nanosecond. All I could do was pray for guidance, and even that required too much effort.

I was so shattered that for the first time in my life I placed my faith in time; it seemed the only potential saving grace available. I felt like I'd been thrown into a wilderness, some harsh, tangled forest of immense suffering. "I can't see the forest through the trees," I told my girlfriends lifelessly. "I finally know what that expression *really* means."

Strangely enough, some part of me knew that things weren't going to get any worse. I knew my soul was meant to arrive here and learn. I was not meant to be with Robert. I was not meant to be with Graham. There was another plan for me, one that I didn't have the will or desire to see right now. But I knew that somewhere up ahead in this dark labyrinthine wilderness, my higher self would find an exit. And she would lead me there.

CHAPTER 3

ONLINE AND OUT OF LINE

Weeks passed. Spring exploded, full of insouciance. And with each passing day, my ice-cold shock began to thaw. As summer came into view, the needs of my kids, their cheer and innocence—even the sun's brilliance against a clean blue sky—made each day progressively bearable. But a part of my chest felt black. Frostbitten. I was maimed yet no one could tell. And the pins and needles of aloneness consumed me. I had no strong arms to hold me. No man to love or make love to me. And no idea of how or if I'd feel passion or bliss ever again. Seriously, what were my options when it came to dating? Go to a bar? Pray that all my married friends would miraculously set me up with a friend? *Pfft.* Not likely. So I remained in stasis, going through the motions of finalizing my divorce and helping the children transition to shared custody. Which they did well. I envied their resilience.

Around this time, my hip pain flared up madly, to the point that I'd be wincing if I rolled on it in my sleep. I had to do something about it and pronto. So I started treatment with a new acupuncturist—this time, a woman. It was through Stephanie that I learned about online dating.

"It's a great alternative to bars," she said enthusiastically, as she swabbed and inserted a pin in my foot. "Especially for busy moms like us who don't have a lot of free time."

"Really?" I replied, surprised. I hadn't even considered online dating. It was like those ads in the back of weeklies that advertised sex calls—somehow it didn't seem quite aboveboard. But if someone like Stephanie used it, apparently it was more mainstream than I thought.

I looked at her more closely. She was in her midthirties, with a few tattoos and streaked blond hair, cut short. "I always thought it sounded kind of creepy," I said skeptically. "Mind you, it wasn't even *invented* when I was last single."

She smiled, not at all offended. "Sure, there're some perverts and weirdoes on there. But you can weed them out. I dated a few really great guys. And one has been my lover now for over a year."

For a second, my body roused to attention; it had been over seven months since I'd made love. But I quickly shoved the feeling back down, irritated with myself. It made no sense to even think about sex, especially when I had urgent responsibilities to tend to, like single parenting.

Stephanie, as if sensing my internal war, leaned into me and gently touched my arm. "Delaine," she said compassionately. "You might be getting divorced, but you aren't dead. You're entitled to have some fun. I remember how hard it was during my divorce. But I vowed there were two things I had to do: find a 'friend with benefits' *and* have sex with a woman." *Wink.* We laughed.

I left her office only mildly interested in the idea of online dating. Besides, who would want to date an older woman like me? Especially one with three young kids? *I'm not ready to date anyway*, I thought to myself.

But now, a dull flash of curiosity got the better of me—and after browsing around on the site she'd recommended, I decided to sign up. "*Pfft.* Why not?" I thought limply.

After selecting a few tasteful photos for my gallery—a casual shot in jeans, a close up where I'm laughing, and a full-body shot of me in a stylish dress—I struggled for over an hour to create a meticulous written profile. It was important to me that I portray myself as a classy woman and devoted mother, the kind of woman a single father and working professional might be attracted to. In no way did I want to seem interested in sex. I didn't even know if I was. But I felt compelled to be prudish, as if my chastity was the prime indicator of my respectability and worth. I had so much to learn.

As an afterthought, I quickly blocked men under the age of thirty-five from contacting me; surely, we'd have nothing in common.

Within minutes of signing up, emails started pouring in, from men of every walk of life. Construction workers, business men, carpenters and college professors—most looked like your average Joe. Some looked downright creepy. A few raised my eyebrow. I sat there glued to my computer, enthralled by the process, astonished that so many men in my age bracket were available, and more importantly, interested in *me*.

Ah, but they sure were looking for different things. Some clearly just wanted to hook up, others were veiled about their intentions (but it was easy to gather that they wanted sex), and others were downright lonely, wanting nothing more than to find a real companion. *I feel you buddy,* I thought more than once. *But you're not my type.* At first, I answered many of the emails out of politeness, but I quickly learned that most guys took this as an invitation. And boy did they come on strong. One guy responded to my brief return email with "10 inches, good and thick, sure you want to pass me up?" *What the?!* Needless to say, it was a fast and dirty learning curve. I went in with no clue to the rules. But I held the reigns. It was liberating to know that I could pick and choose who I responded to.

Days turned to weeks, and the mail kept flowing in. I now had a new hobby, one that stroked my ego and temporarily pulled me out of my ennui. It was positive reinforcement on steroids, and like an addict, I checked my email throughout the day. At eight 'o clock, when lights were out, kids in bed, I'd lock myself in my office for the rest of the evening—reading, searching, replying . . . At this point, I'd even begun flirting with a few: "Dear Stuart, you flatter me, but I could say the same about you. You look as hot as you are smart . . ." Communicating by email felt so safe and nonthreatening, I found that in this suspended reality, I could set all my pain and loneliness aside and be candid and flirty, daring or thoughtful, without rebuke or self-consciousness. It was empowering.

It became so all-consuming that come morning, as soon as my kids were fed, I'd race downstairs in my slippers and log on again. I even checked my mail in the middle of the night. God, how I hated the night hours. If and when sleep finally found me, I'd often wake up worrying—no, *panicking*—about my life, ruminating over my past, my body cold with stress. It seemed I could divert myself during the day, but whenever I tried to sleep, my subconscious mind went into overdrive, desperately seeking answers, frantic to help me chart a True North again.

So instead of lying in bed, deluged by melancholy and playing the same mental tapes over and over again, I would put on my housecoat, go to my computer, and log on.

FINALLY, I AGREED to meet a man from the dating site. His name was Cal, and he apparently worked in executive management. At thirty-seven, he was also separated with two kids. Through our *fifty* email exchanges, where I'd bombarded him with questions, I'd deduced that he was a family man, a man with strong values, the kind of man a woman in my position should date. It also didn't hurt that he was pretty good looking, too: clean shaven with sandy brown hair and intense hazel eyes.

I sat in the coffee shop with my eyes glued to the front entrance. I was a bundle of nerves. This was a huge step for me—my first real date in over a decade—and my first foray out with a man since Graham. My stomach wouldn't let me forget it. It helped that I felt confident about how I looked: My dark jeans and fuchsia wrap-shirt accentuated my slim figure; and my hair, which I wore loose and wavy down my back, had been freshly highlighted. My freckled skin looked healthy and clear, with minimal makeup, and I'd applied a fresh coat of lipgloss in the car. *Good to go . . .*

As I sat there clenching and unclenching my tea mug, I worried, *Oh, what if he's unattractive?* His profile said he was six-foot-three and 240 pounds. I'd never been out with a man that big before. Robert and Graham were both over six feet tall but on the slender side—that's what I was used to, so that's what I preferred. But Cal said he was a former defenseman in the pro hockey league. Surely he must be muscular. *God I hope he isn't fat,* I thought, and then I quickly chastised myself. *Do I really even want to do this . . . ?*

Fifteen minutes later, he still hadn't shown. I began to panic. *Am I to be stood up on my first date?* I thought. *Well that's just great . . .*

Elbows deep in my purse, I was scrambling to find his phone number when a giant-sized man in an elegant grey suit lumbered into the cafe. He walked right up to me and offered me his big hand and a smile. "Hi, Delaine," he said. *Deep voice. Nice.* "I'm Cal. I'm so sorry I'm late. I had to park about ten blocks down the street. I'm just going to run to the bathroom, okay?"

"No problem," I said, sneaking a long peek at him as he walked away. I shifted my purse onto the vacant chair beside me and smiled. Thumbs up to him being attractive, polished, and very masculine. My nervousness turned into excitement.

Two minutes later, he crouched into the wooden chair across

from me. *Groan*, belched the chair, responding to his weight. I suppressed a laugh and pretended not to notice.

"So," he said casually, a warm smile on his face. "This is the first time you've met someone from the site, eh?"

"Yes."

"Are you nervous?"

"A little." I'd unknowingly grabbed the tea bag package and was tearing it into little pieces.

"Don't worry. I promise I don't bite." He leaned back in his chair, hands interlocked behind his head, when all of a sudden, the little wooden legs let out a God-awful, *CREAK!* This time, we both laughed.

Our conversation flowed easily from there—work, friends, our kids, dating. But still, I kept reminding myself to speak confidently. *He doesn't know about your past, nor does he need to. Just think of this as a job interview.*

Our meeting lasted only forty-five minutes; he had to get back to his office. But it was enough. I liked his smile, I liked his energy, and I could tell he liked mine; I swear his pupils were dilated. I felt the physical connection too: such enormous shoulders, such wide playful lips, such massive knuckles . . .

I *knew* I would see this man again.

A FEW NIGHTS later, I nervously primped for our second date. My body tingled with anticipation, but my brain was wrought with worry. I didn't know what the rules for dating and having sex were anymore. Should I avoid falling into bed with him at all costs, even at my age? What if I couldn't emotionally handle having sex again? What if the sex was awful, even worse than it was with Robert, and I found myself going through the motions with a stranger I cared nothing about? And most disturbing yet annoying of all: What if he didn't like my body? I'd struggled my entire teenage and adult life not to buy into society's negative messages around age and beauty. But the truth was that I held the shoppers Optimum card. Even with Graham, who openly admired my body, I was still self-conscious. Three pregnancies and childbirths had left battle scars as souvenirs: my breasts were lower, my stomach flabbier, a C-section scar highlighted my pubic bone. *When does the body image war ever end?* I wondered, irritated. These scars should be badges of honor, not markings of shame.

For this date, we planned to meet at a popular upscale bar and restaurant. And I planned to trade in my tea cup for a wine glass. Due to my back-to-back pregnancies, I had a very low tolerance for alcohol; my friends called me the One-Glass Wonder. But tonight I *wanted* to loosen up.

As we sat amongst the busy crowd of men and women, many still wearing suits from work, it struck me how this whole "adult world" had ticked along during my ten-year retreat to the suburban universe. It felt exhilarating to be a part of it again, and the mood helped me relax into conversation with Cal.

But somewhere midway through my second glass of wine and his third beer, our sexual attraction started hindering the conversation. We'd hold each other's gaze, our sentences going unfinished, as we silently wandered up and down each other's body. Finally, he took the initiative and sat down beside me. He covered my thigh with his hand and I grabbed it, squeezed it, inviting him to feel and know me more. I couldn't think, I couldn't even talk; every nerve-ending in my body was on fire.

"Let's get out of here," he murmured, his voice husky. I nodded.

We walked briskly to his condo three blocks away. I feigned interest in his décor, which was a mix of modern chic and masculine simplicity, while he turned on some jazzy background music and dimmed the lights. Suddenly he was looming over me. He pinned me against the wall, kissing me hard. My body blossomed under the taste and power of his lips and the feel of his huge strong body against mine. He could snap me in half if he wanted to, but he knew his own strength. It was intensely arousing. He spun me around, pressing my face and body into the wall, his large hands eagerly moving all over me. The strength and ownership in his touch left me unable to think, unable to doubt what I was doing—oh the pleasure, the hunger, the rawness of my need. He picked me up and carried me to the kitchen. Somewhere along the way, he removed his clothes *and* mine. He lifted me on to the counter, my legs pressed round his hips, and for the first time in eight months I allowed a man to have me, and me him. The moment he entered me, I felt nothing but desire—and entitlement. *I* wanted this. My body wanted this . . . We were heat and passion, and then he carried me to the couch and we explored each other in numerous positions. He carried me to his bedroom, but not before we lingered in the hall. He pressed his lips against my ears, his breath hot, and talked dirty to me, his words and his deep voice flooding me with arousal. "You're so fucking wet, I could cum right now," he said, groaning into my ear. "But I'm not. Oh no, I'm going to . . . " He lead, I followed, willingly, ardently, my body on fire.

I was straddling him on his queen-size bed when he finished. He shuddered and moaned, and I knew he'd orgasmed hard. I lay forward onto his chest, which was slick with sweat, both of us breathing hard. My arms and legs trembled, even though I hadn't climaxed. But I was okay with that. The tornado of what just transpired felt like one giant climax. Besides, it wasn't fair to expect him to understand my body during our first encounter. His hands gently caressed my back, and a calm, comfortable silence enveloped us. I nuzzled my head into the crevice between his shoulder and neck and closed my eyes.

And that's when the tears came. Surprising and unexpected.

I fought to stop them. I knew my body was feeling and wanting to tell me something, but c'mon—*NOW?*

"Hey," Cal gently asked, "Are you okay?"

"Yeah . . . I'm just a bit emotional, that's all. It's been a long time."

He hugged me tenderly. "*Shhh* . . . it's okay." I carefully rolled off of him and snuggled into his chest. He continued touching me gently—my arms, my back—and my silent tears trickled down my face in the darkness.

It felt so good to be touched again, to be held in the strong, comforting arms of a man. I had waited and waited so long for Graham. I had longed and ached for his touch and embrace with every part of my body and soul. And now, lying naked in this stranger's arms, a wave of emotions swelled to life inside of me. I felt vulnerable and raw; *alive.* Having sex again had pushed vital life energy throughout my entire body, which had felt dead for so long. Sex had made me go inside this tomb and *feel.* And as I lay there with Cal, the concentrated energy in my heart began pressing against my throat: I was either going to sob uncontrollably or talk. The gates were opening and I couldn't stop them.

So I told him. I told him in less than a minute about Robert and Graham's betrayals. My affair with Graham was something I'd sworn I'd never tell another man, if not for the humiliation but for the shame of it. But here it was anyway. I even told him about the baby. I confessed that I was still in love with Graham and my heart was broken. At that point, I got up, dressed, and left.

I walked back to the bar knowing I had just made a complete fool out of myself. Talk about ruining a date! But I didn't care. All I could think about was Graham. I got in my car and drove to his house. I was crying and smoked three cigarettes along the way. Tonight was the night I was going to show Graham my pain. He deserved to see the aftermath of his choices. He deserved to witness this pile of rubble called Delaine.

I walked to his door and rang his doorbell. It was 1:00 AM. He didn't answer, so I rang it again. And again. But the lights were out and his truck wasn't parked in the driveway. I knew he wasn't home, but I continued to stand there anyway, crying, pacing, and peering in through the windows like a stalker. I knew I was being saved the total humiliation of what I was doing. I knew I was acting like a crazy woman. But I didn't care. I was tired of being the bigger person! To just forgive his selfish, stupid, cruel behavior. *I'm not a fucking angel! I'm a flesh and blood, passionate, caring, FEELING woman. And I'm sick of putting everyone else's feelings before mine, I'm entitled to some hysterics, and Goddamnit, I say it's going to happen right now!*

I slumped down on his porch with my arms covering my head. I rocked back and forth, as my rage and anguish settled in for the kill.

Ten minutes later, I got back in my car and quickly drove away, followed by one cogent thought.

Thank God no one saw me!

CHAPTER 4

FRIENDS IN NEED

"YOU DID *WHAT*?" MY BEST friend Hali exclaimed over the phone. "Why the hell did you go to Graham's house?"

It was the next morning and I felt plain terrible. But I didn't want to get into it, since it wasn't an appropriate time: Hali was due to give birth to her second child in a few weeks, and me and our closest girlfriends were throwing her a baby shower in a few hours.

"I don't know . . . I guess having sex with Cal triggered stuff," I offered wearily.

"And . . . How was it?" she asked.

"How was what?"

"*Sex with Cal!*"

Erotic snapshots flashed through my mind. I couldn't fight off a grin. "It was fun. Really fun, actually. But I'm sure he thinks I'm a psycho. I cried after we had sex *and* I told him about Graham and the baby. He probably can't run far enough away from me."

"Oh Delaine!" I knew she was shaking her head. "Well, at least you finally had sex again. You've now gotten the 'first time' over with and that's a big deal. I'm sure it'll help you move on faster."

"Let's hope so," I said. "Anyway, moving on to your baby shower, I'll be arriving at your place an hour early. I've a few games and things to set up."

"Awesome, I'll see you soon."

For the next hour, I focused on the final preparations for Hali's shower. More than anything I wanted today's celebration to be *extra* special for Hali, not only because she deserved it, but because she *needed* it.

At three months pregnant, Hali discovered that her husband, Paul, was having an affair. She'd accidentally stumbled across a peculiar email, and when she casually approached him about it, he crumbled instantly. In tears, his rugged chin down, he begged her to understand that he was in love with this other woman. He believed they were "soul mates"; how could he walk away from her, the "love of his life"? He was just "so confused and lost. Couldn't she see that? Where was her compassion?" And with that, he abandoned his stunned, horrified, pregnant wife and four-year-old son to go "find himself"—and his girlfriend.

As Hali dealt with the aftermath of betrayal—not sleeping, not eating, emotionally floundering and flailing—I was there for her. I babysat her son whenever possible to give her time to rest and grieve. I listened when she called, teary, at 2:00 AM, needing courage and compassion and commiseration. Even though I was still seeing Graham at the time, I understood her. I'd gone through it with Robert. Little did I know that in a few months, I'd be in her shoes— again—and while the irony was not lost on me that I was "the other woman," Hali never judged me. It helped that both Graham's marriage and my own had ended, if not literally, then emotionally. Hali and I each, in our separate and similar ways, understood the scorching pain of deceit and heartbreak. We were both forced to sift through the ashes of our family dreams for a new foundation. Life was tough. We couldn't have needed each other more.

Despite it all, Hali not only "got through" the next six months of her pregnancy, she did so with a toughness and determination that belied her inner despair. She immediately began hashing through the legalities of their separation, moved into their just-completed dream house without him, constructed new dreams as a single mom-to-be of two children, *and* planned a home birth. I admired her deeply. In my eyes, she was the embodiment of a powerful woman.

Hali's shower was a marvelous success. I'm not sure which was stronger: Hali's glow or the amount of warmth and laughter in her house. Either way, I knew she was basking in and absorbing the loving energy we'd created. So, too, were the freshly painted walls of her brand new, albeit single-mom, home.

"I'VE BEEN FEELING kind of funny all morning," said Hali, gently rubbing her giant belly. "I kind of think today might be the day."

We were sitting in the shopping mall food court having lunch. She was due any day, so I packed the kids in the minivan and joined her on a last-minute foray for baby gear. As we sat finishing our lunches, we kept an eye on the kids as they monkeyed in the atrium.

I looked at Hali closely. She looked radiant.

"Yep. You're ready," I concluded.

"I *am*," she said, patting her belly and smiling. "I am ready to meet my daughter.

"You know what Delaine?" she continued, picking at her salad. "As exciting as it is that I'll soon meet my daughter, I also can't wait to get back out there and start dating again." She leaned in conspiratorially, looking around to make sure no one was listening. "I *really* want to have sex again. I mean seriously, it's been a long six months."

"I *know* it has," I said laughing. "Remember how you wanted to go speed dating when you first found out about Paul's affair? You were three months pregnant, for God's sake!"

"Crazy, eh?" she laughed. "But I wanted to do it while I could still hide my pregnancy."

I shook my head, "That is crazy, hon. I'm glad you didn't do it."

She smiled, but her eyes suddenly turned more serious. "It just hasn't been fair. Paul freely spent these past six months feeling giddy-in-love with someone new, while I was left to pick up the pieces, look after the kids, and go through all of this alone. I've wanted so badly to lean on another man, to have someone tell me I'm desirable and lovable. But instead I've had to give that comfort to myself. Hell, I couldn't even turn to alcohol or smoking to make me feel better!"

I listened, seeing the weight of her burdens and loneliness shift across her face.

"I know all this was supposed to make me stronger," she continued, raising her chin. "It *has* made me stronger, but I swear to God," she added passionately, "as soon as the midwives give me the thumbs up, I'm going to find me a well-hung man and screw the hell out of him!"

I laughed, full bellied, at the powerful irony of what she'd just said. Visions of happily married pregnant moms gasping raced through my mind.

"So what's happening with you and Cal?" she asked.

Despite my post-sex dramatics, Cal *did* contact me again, and we'd met up afterward for a few more sweaty trysts.

"I like him. He's a nice guy," I said, shrugging. "But I just don't see it going anywhere."

"Why does it have to *go* anywhere? The sex is good, isn't it?"

"Sure. It's okay," I said. Now it was my turn to lean in a little closer and ensure young ears were out of reach. "I mean, I like the way we have sex—he picks me up a lot and is very aggressive, which is fun—but I've never had an orgasm with him. And well, I hate to be mean, but . . . *his penis is really quite small.*"

Hali burst out laughing. "Really? Like how small? What *is* small, anyway? I've just never had an issue with that."

"I don't know exact measurements," I said, grinning. "But let's put it this way: When I put my hand around him, I easily cover him from top to bottom."

"Hmmmm," Hali said, trying not to laugh. "Not good."

"*Pfft*, tell me about it! I mean, if he was into oral sex or he was more sensual, then perhaps it wouldn't bother me. But he's so physical. *Sexual*, not sensual. He fucks like a hockey player." I lifted my elbows and shoulders. "Like an NHL fighter." Hali laughed and I joined in.

"Anyway," I said, shaking my head. "We'll see what happens. I'm not writing Cal off or anything—"

"No, you're just keeping keep him around till a guy with a bigger penis comes along!"

I laughed and pushed my chair back. "Let's go run these monsters through the mall. I promised the boys they could look at light sabers at Toys"R"Us, too.

"Sounds good," she said.

But our shopping expedition didn't last long: Hali suddenly began having contractions, and within half an hour, she was leaning on the wall breathing hard. It was time to go.

Two DAYS LATER, Cal and I had a disagreement and that marked the end of our brief tryst. We had different perspectives about dating. Even though we weren't in a serious relationship, he didn't want me to stay active on the dating site, and my feelings for him weren't strong enough to do that.

While my interest in Cal was casual at best, the fallout hit me surprisingly hard. I was still more fragile than I believed. I had mistaken emotional numbness for healing, not self-protection. I was back in that forest, unsure where the path was—or if one even existed. I had no road map, no compass, no idea of what my future would hold, and I had this unnerving sense that I didn't know who

I was anymore. How would I manage being a single mother of three and how would I support us financially? What if I never again found the kind of love I'd felt with Graham? I still couldn't see the forest for the trees. I retreated, without resistance, into the shadows of self-pity. I didn't realize that I could manage my life alone.

Fueled by my angst, over the next eight weeks of summer I met twelve different men from the dating site. I wasn't just dating "anyone." I still screened them carefully and adhered to my original age and job requirements. But unconsciously, my mission was clear: Seek and Replace.

The problem was, there wasn't a single man I wanted to see beyond a first coffee date. I simply wasn't attracted to any of them. But in place of desire, something else was surfacing. Something I *needed*, something I was grateful for. The seedlings of confidence.

"WHAT WAS WRONG with the last guy, the skinny guy in the convertible?" asked Hali. She and her kids were over for a playdate, and we were sitting in my sunny kitchen, drinking tea. Hali's daughter, Teah, was now six weeks old, and Hali, true to her word, was dating again, too.

I grinned over my teacup. "I liked him, and we got along well. But at the end of our date, he kissed me. And well . . ." I scrunched up my nose. "He gave my face a bath."

Hali laughed, then said, "Hmmm. A kiss is important. Maybe he was just nervous?"

"I considered that. So I let him kiss me again. But nope, same thing."

"Yuck. Well that's no good. If he can't get a kiss right, don't risk finding out what he's inept at in bed."

"Moooom!" My three-year-old daughter suddenly hollered from down in the basement. *"Evan said I'm a stupid dummy."*

I rolled my eyes. "Ah, the joys of parenting . . ." I got up and went to the foot of the stairs. My five-year-old, Evan, was bursting to proclaim his innocence. "Listen up guys: Evan, there will be no name-calling. And that goes for the rest of you, too. Play nice or I'll separate you."

"*Yes mom*," came their voices in unison.

I sat back down at the table. "Let's see how long *that* lasts."

Hali grinned. "Anyhow," she began again. "I find it strange that you've met so many men and rejected them all. Maybe if you got to know them better, someone would grow on you."

"Believe me Hali. I *want* to like these guys. My *body* wants me to like these guys. I wish I wasn't so damn picky." I shook my head in frustration. "But something kind of positive *has* actually come out of all this serial dating . . ."

Hali raised her brows. "What's that?"

"When I first started meeting men, and someone would give me a compliment like, 'You're so funny,' or 'You're so smart and interesting,' I couldn't believe they were talking about me. I literally sat there going, *huh*? I wasn't able to fully receive the compliments, as if there was a big wall there. But now I'm starting to internalize them a bit. And wow, it feels pretty darn good."

"Well *I* can tell you why you've had trouble believing their compliments," Hali said adamantly. "It's because you were married for seven years to a bully who constantly put you down. He ridiculed you *constantly* Delaine, even in front of all your friends. I'd sit there growing angrier and angrier, just waiting for you to stick up for yourself. But you just laughed it off. *Grrr,* I get worked up just thinking about it. Thank God you're divorcing him."

"But . . . I—"

"And don't get me started on Graham!" she said, cutting me off. She was on a roll. "You said he was so wonderful. You always said you had no idea he was having an affair. But did he call you when he said he would? *No.* Did he make an extra effort to see you? *No.* Did he show you in a thousand ways that he thought you were the most amazing woman on earth? *Not even close*. That's not love."

"Okay, okay! Uncle, already," I said, even though I didn't think Hali's assessment was fair. Hali hadn't seen how he treated me when we were together—how attentive he was, how he looked at me, how he laughed and shared and showered me with his love. The possibility of him cheating with a second woman had never crossed my mind!

"Let's not go there, okay hon? I'm all about trying to move forward. Speaking of which, what about that guy you accidentally met on your date the other day?" Only Hali could go out on her first date in thirteen years, go to the wrong place, and pick up a *different* man while she waited.

"Josh? Oh, it's nothing really. I just gave him my number. I enjoyed talking to him, but in all honesty, I had trouble understanding him. He's from Newfoundland and his accent is really thick."

"How old is he?"

"Thirty-three. And he's *not* good looking. I mean, he's okay, but he's nothing special. God, listen to me, eh? That sounds terrible. Anyway, he might be someone I can hang out with . . . or maybe even have *sex* with," she added, smiling coyly. "We'll see."

Suddenly, Teah started stirring in her car seat. As Hali got up to prepare her bottle, I couldn't help but admire how pretty she looked: Her blue satin blouse complemented her skin and blond hair, and from behind, she looked sexy in her stylish, hip-hugging blue jeans. "By the way, you really look fantastic, hon," I said.

"Thanks. I feel pretty good about how I look. But you know me—there's always a battle raging with body image. Look at this—" She lifted her shirt and squeezed the soft skin around her waist. "See? Mommy belly. It's so obvious. And I worry that any man I sleep with will get stuck on the fact that I recently gave birth.

"If he has a problem with it, it's his. You gave birth only six weeks ago! Your stomach is *supposed* to look like that."

"I know I know," she grumbled as she tested the milk on her wrist. "I'm also really worried about being too 'loose' down there. *Pfft*. As if dating again wasn't challenge enough."

"Just keep kegeling, hon. Do it for the sake of continence first and foremost. Said by a woman who's given birth to three! Besides, at the end of the day, when it comes to sex, I think most men are just happy to have it."

We each sat quietly for a moment, watching Teah as she drank her bottle. "I still can't believe this is our life right now," murmured Hali, gently rocking her daughter. "I just never, *ever*, would have imagined myself going through all of this."

"I know," I said, shaking my head. "Isn't it wild that we're going through this at the exact same time?"

"Yeah . . . But I know that a year from now, our lives will look completely different. *Way better.*"

"WAY better," I said, nodding. I then added thoughtfully: "I remember an older lady once saying to me, 'Every woman goes through a period of insanity at some point in her life.' Not as in 'she loses her mind' or she 'caves to hysteria' but that life tests her so hard that she's forced to question and own and grow into all that she can be.

"And you know what, Hali? There's no doubt in my mind that we're right in the thick of ours."

CHAPTER 5

AFTERNOON DELIGHT

IT WAS THE FIRST TIME Robert had ever taken the children on a weekend instead of midweek. Better still, it was a long weekend. Elated with my newfound freedom, I spent the latter part of Friday night glued to my computer, trawling the online dating site; this *had* to be the weekend where I'd find a meaningful relationship.

By 2:00 AM, I had no real prospects; a few potentials though: a cute electrician from a neighboring city, a divorced dad with three kids. Normal guys, average looking, but missing something all the same. *Hopefully tomorrow,* I thought optimistically, as I climbed into bed.

Early Saturday morning I quickly signed in at my desk and sorted through my inbox. A few men had responded to my inquiries, but still, nobody looked promising. My body gushed with sensual agitation. I yearned to feel a man's hands on me. Not just yearned, *craved.* Every nerve ending was alive with need, and the clock was ticking down the weekend. *Dammit, Delaine, look harder!*

But I was struggling with competing desires. I dropped my face into my hands. I couldn't just go have sex with any "body." The physicality of sex alone wasn't enough for me—I knew too well from marriage that body parts "getting satisfied" could feel empty, even gross. Sure, that hadn't happened with Cal, but maybe I just got lucky. No. I couldn't risk it. Above all, I needed connection. Respect. Because of my relationship with Graham, I knew what it felt like to make love. If I couldn't look into a man's eyes or talk with him for hours afterward, at least as a close friend, why bother? I'd be selling myself short; I'd be moving backwards.

But my body was screaming for sex. It was affecting my mood. I couldn't concentrate on anything. I was uptight, irritable, and only a marathon of fevered, animalistic sex would pacify me.

At that moment, the sexual energy that Graham had unleashed in me felt like both a blessing and a curse. I was thrilled to know I wasn't sexually dead, like I had been during my marriage. But all that concentrated energy seemed to be pooling and leaking into my brain; it was taking on a life force of its own, and I didn't know what to do with it.

My thoughts jumped impatiently to Hali and her new lover, Josh. Soon after their accidental meeting in the bar, she'd taken him to bed—despite the fact that she wasn't very attracted to him, despite the fact that he wasn't relationship potential. But Hali quickly recognized his other merits: he stroked her ego and made her feel good about her body. Moreover, he was well endowed *and* regularly supplied her with sensational orgasms.

I was happy for her. Taking another lover after thirteen years of marriage was a huge deal. But I was also envious. Here she was, barely two months postpartum, having only dated for a couple of weeks, and already "getting some." No, not "some"—she was getting *lots*. Cal and I had sex only three times, I hadn't orgasmed at all, and he had a penis the size of a thumb. Why was this taking so long for me? Why did I have so many rules and expectations—of me *and* the men I dated?

I so rarely get time off to myself, I'm sure as heck not going to waste it, I thought determinedly, as I picked up the phone and called my longtime friend Patty.

Patty was my older totally striking single girlfriend. I didn't know her exact age, but I'd wager somewhere in her midfifties, even though she looked ten years younger. Petite, exotic looking, with ample breasts, she made men, young and old, do triple takes when she walked into a room.

"Hey, Delaine!" she said warmly. "How *are* you?"

"Not good, Patty. I need your help."

I explained my situation to her, no candy coating required. "I feel like I'm going crazy, Patty; sex is all I can think about. But I have all these *rules*, these stupid, ridiculous rules in my head about what I should and shouldn't do. But . . . today I'm feeling wild and irresponsible. I keep telling myself I need a *relationship* and it has to be with a man over thirty-five. But *screw* it. Today I'm lifting the restrictions."

"You want me to find you a young man," she said matter-of-factly. "Yes!" I said, relieved that she got it. I felt emboldened. "I want a hot young man to come to my house, preferably one with a large penis, and have him screw the heck out of me. It'll be a one-time thing only." *WHAT? Have you lost your mind?*

She laughed, but knowingly. "I know a guy who'd be *perfect* for you." Give me a few minutes and I'll phone you back."

Half an hour later I was frantically pulling garments from my lingerie drawer—a hot twenty-seven-year-old was on his way over! What to wear? What do I feel sexy in? How does a woman even *dress* for this?

I decided on a black, lacy bra and matching panties—simple, sophisticated, sexy. My breasts looked perky and full; tummy, relatively flat from not eating and smoking too many cigarettes last night. *I look good. I am a sexy woman. And unless he takes a close look at my skin, he'll never know I have three kids. Hmm . . . hold on a second, if I end up on top he's going to see saggy Momma Belly.* I quickly reached up and closed my window blinds to the max.

Wearing black stilettos and a short satin housecoat, I clip-clopped over to the bathroom mirror. Lips looked full, freckled skin clear and smudge-free, no boogers hanging out, dirty-blond hair curly and luxuriously long. I didn't look like I was twenty-five—my crow's feet made that impossible. *But I'm a damn good thirty-seven*, I said to myself. And I'm *entitled* to do this. Everyone in the world might call me a tramp right now, but I don't care! They're mistaken: I am a Woman Entitled.

But what about the kids' rooms?

I clattered down my bungalow hallway and shut their bed-room doors, not before admonishing myself for their messiness. *Don't think about that now!* Right now, I am not Delaine the Mom, I am Delaine the Vixen, the Seduction Goddess, a woman who demands and receives what she wants.

Back up the hall, I stood by the front door. I told him exactly what I wanted: that he was to just walk in; that he wasn't to talk to me. I would be ready and waiting for him. No other details were required.

Oh, but I couldn't stand THERE, it looked too contrived, and I felt like an idiot! I moved back a few steps, slightly around the corner. *Much better.*

What if he thinks I look fat? What if he thinks I look old? I'll KNOW it—I'll see it on his face.

Oh get a grip on yourself! I screamed in my head. *You look hot, this entire scenario is hot, so step up, and for God's sake, shut up!*

I leaned against the wall, hearing only the sultry music of Fiona Apple coming from my bedroom and my heart hammering in my ears. The squeak of the doorknob turned; a tall, hunky, dark-haired man in blue jeans and T-shirt entered, looked around, and saw me: two strangers meeting for the first time. He quickly slipped off his shoes and took me in with his eyes. He walked toward me, a moment frozen in time. All that mattered was *right now.*

Suddenly, his lips were on my ear: "You are *so* hot," he whispered, his breath tickling my skin. Desire shot through me—ferocious, yearning. I placed my arms around his neck and felt his big hands slide under my housecoat across my naked back. I opened my body to him . . . and kissed him passionately.

Down the hall he carried me, my legs wrapped around his hips, our lips never parting. As we stood at the foot of my bed, I looked up into his unfamiliar face and thought, *Oh, he has a crooked nose.* But as he pulled off his shirt, my eyes beheld such yumminess that all conscious thinking was decimated by lust.

I have to admit, Yummy Stranger's sexual skills were pretty novice. I had to take control and show him what to do, especially to achieve the orgasm I desperately wanted. He knew where to find my clit with his fingers, but the motion, the pressure he applied, was way off. I reached down and began guiding his hand with my own, whispering and directing him with my words and moans. Moreover, not to dwell on this point—or this part of a man's anatomy—but his penis was on the small size, too. *Does* penis size and shape matter? Ask ten different women and you might get ten different answers, including: "What a shallow thing to ask." *My* honest answer is, "Maybe . . . still under investigation!" I'd never realized before how different men are in terms of size and aesthetics. I'd experienced numerous partners before getting married, but back then, I was so preoccupied with the emotional side of sex, that I didn't dare analyze the merits or shortcomings of my partner's tackle. All I knew was that today, had Yummy Stranger been well- and beautifully-endowed, I would have been *delighted.* Morally right or wrong, I think I had a new appreciation developing.

Once Yummy Stranger and I finished and we lay in my joyfully disheveled bed, catching our breaths, I felt rather awkward. I'd just gotten naked with someone I knew nothing about. *Now what?* Good manners prompted me to start making casual conversation, but then I stopped. Truly, why bother? Instead, I laughed and said, "Thanks, that was fun. Hope you enjoy the rest of your day." He quickly took his cue to get up, get dressed, and get out. I didn't even walk him to the door.

I wondered: *Did I just treat him disrespectfully? Was that rude? Mean? Degrading?*

No, I decided. I had been honest from the get-go about what I wanted. We had fulfilled our deal and then it was over. Like I tell my kids at a playdate, "Every playdate has a beginning and an end. When the end comes, put on your jacket, say thank you, and go home." My afternoon rendezvous was an "adult playdate"—I expected no tantrums or upset feelings, thanks very much.

Still, I marveled at how I felt no need to cuddle or get to know him. He was just a scrumptious, young body. I felt and wanted no mental or emotional connection with him. I didn't want to talk to him and explain why I had invited him over. I didn't want to justify or explain *anything* to him. Why should I? He would never know or understand me. He was simply the character in my fantasy. Yes, this was a fantasy. *And really,* I thought with relish, smiling, *he was lucky to have been a part of it.* How many young men only dream of spending an impromptu afternoon of uninhibited sex with a sexy, older woman?

I rolled over on my side and closed my eyes. My pillow felt so comfy . . . I was glad to be cuddling with it and not him. Post-orgasm fatigue descended on me.

THE NEXT DAY, I felt downright giddy about my illicit afternoon. Maybe *too* great. Was my behavior slutty? Was it but one more sign that my life, my character, was spiraling hellward fast? Did I need to be slapped, thrashed, or verbally dragged back across the border to Good Girl Land?

These were questions for the girlfriends. But *select* girlfriends. Only the most nonjudgmental and liberated. But Hali, my first choice, was busy with her kids. Who else might be free for a weekend powwow lunch?

As I mentally scanned through my "mom friends"—the ones I saw regularly in my community—my mind drifted to a recent gathering we'd shared at a local pub. That night, all the ladies had expressed both concern and curiosity over my transition to single life. I didn't tell them very much. I did tell them about Cal, the hockey defenseman, minus all the (small penis) details, of course. And I told them about the wacky world of online dating and how I'd met "a few" men off there for coffee. My mom friends listened *very* attentively. And whenever I stopped talking, someone would quickly insert another dating question. When the questions finally stopped, an intense dead air loomed above the table.

"I just don't know what else to talk about," my friend Diane finally exhaled. "Our lives just sound so boring."

I realized that night that I was experiencing something beyond these ladies' reference frame. They were all still married and focused on their careers and families. The entire time I spoke at our table, a voice kept whispering in my ear, *Be careful what you say. They care about you, but they don't understand, and they are JUDG-ING you.*

Ultimately, I believed the scope of people's empathy and support did, in large part, stem from their own personal experiences. And let's face it, experience—a casual, afternoon romp with a yummy young stranger—wasn't one many women my age would relate to. Especially my married mom friends. They'd probably downright disapprove. Yet I totally understood why: My current escapades simply did not blend with their family-oriented looking glass on life; they contradicted it. Insulted it. Maybe even tested it. I just knew I had to be careful who I told about my experiences. One wrong set of ears, and I'd be headline news on the school playground.

Luckily, my close and longtime non-mom friends, Tory and her sister, Shiloh, were free for an impromptu tête-à-tête. I blurted out my entire story, no censorship required, before the waitress even served our drinks.

"I think your rendezvous sounds empowering," Tory said, matter-of-factly.

"Honestly? You don't think I should feel guilty?"

"Delaine, you had sex on *your* terms," she said firmly. "You're a grown woman and you're entitled to some fun. Your story actually reminds me of the wild things I did when I was dating years ago."

I watched as Tory dropped her chin and giggled, blue eyes peering up through her bob-cut blond hair. She continued: "I remember once, when I was twenty, I went to pick up my boyfriend at the train station wearing nothing but a trench coat and high heels. It was so exciting to walk around at the train station knowing I was naked underneath, knowing I would blow his mind. But then his train was two hours late. *And* it was minus-thirty outside. I darn near froze my butt off!"

As we laughed, I could easily picture Tory doing such a thing. We'd lived together for a while back in our twenties, and let's just say the wall between our bedrooms was a little thin. On the outside, she came across as being sweet and innocent, and I'd watched men flock to her like bears on honey. But behind closed doors, a hungry tigress was unleashed. Guys must have thought they'd died and gone to heaven. Now, at thirty-eight, successful in her career, comfortable in her own skin and happily married, I trusted and respected her deeply.

"I did some pretty wild sexy things when I was younger too," I reflected. "But there's a big difference between what I did back then versus what I did yesterday." Tory looked at me attentively. "Those sexy scenarios from my younger days were mainly designed to please the *man*. On some level, sure, I was having fun too. But ultimately, I was using my sexual prowess as a weapon: to win him, to keep him, to make him love me. It came from a place of insecurity.

"But yesterday's meeting was not about him, not in the least. Sure, I wanted him to have fun too, but my primary objective was to satisfy myself. I decided I wanted sex, I decided where, how and with whom, and I felt mentally and emotionally entitled to have it as I pleased."

It felt good to admit this, to own up to my newfound conviction, which felt fresh and liberating. It was a good feeling—no, not just good. *Great.*

"I get you," Tory said thoughtfully. "There *is* a big difference. It *was* mainly about the man back then. How many times did we put up with men being selfish in bed? How many times did they orgasm and we didn't? And we just accepted it. We women are trained to be so darn polite."

"And how many times in the aftermath did they not want to cuddle or spend the night like we wanted?" I added. "That's why it felt kind of good to push him out the door. It felt like role reversal."

I paused as the waitress served our food. "In a way, the whole thing almost feels imagined now. It was like some wild persona came over me; I was me . . . and yet, I wasn't me." I shook my head trying to understand. "I keep thinking I should feel bad about myself for what I did. I almost WANT to feel bad about myself so that I'll know I have some morals. But the truth is, every time I think of it, I can't stop smiling."

"Well *I* think you have every right to smile," Shiloh piped in, having listened quietly up until now.

Tory laughed. "Of course you do! You're having sex with two different guys."

"You *are*?" I said with surprise. I still thought of Shiloh as being so young and innocent, even though she was twenty-five. It seemed like just yesterday she was fifteen and telling me about losing her virginity. Now, as I gazed at this poised, dark-eyed woman across from me, I realized it was time to get current. "How did this happen?" I asked. "Do they know about each other?"

"No. I met them off a dating site, too," Shiloh said, pushing strands of her long, curly hair away from her face. "Until the 'exclusivity' conversation comes up, you're free to date and have sex with whomever you please."

I was flabbergasted. I thought *my* generation of women was sexually liberated, yet here she was already doing what I'd never done before.

"That's the way it works today," Shiloh explained. "So I have one guy who I enjoy spending time with—he's really sweet and the sex is okay. And one other guy—Rocko *(laugh)*—who I call just for wild, passionate sex."

Tory, seeing the shocked look on my face, jumped in: "Dating has changed a lot since we were younger, Delaine. I hear Shiloh's stories and one thing's for sure, things move a *lot* faster than they did before. The rules are whatever you make them."

OUTSIDE THE RESTAURANT, I had just said goodbye to the girls when I remembered I owed Tory money for a girls' trip to Las Vegas she was organizing. I caught up to her on the sidewalk, gave her a check and another hug goodbye.

Vegas. I couldn't believe it. It was the ultimate fabulous cliché trip for any group of women to take, and I couldn't be more delighted. A couple of months after the Graham bomb went off, I kept feeling the need to get away; escape. "How about Vegas?" I threw out to my girlfriends one afternoon, when we'd met for lunch. "I've never been there before. Anyone want to come?" I crossed my fingers that one or two would be free; we'd tried to organize such trips in the past, but careers, kids, or some life variable always choked our plans. It seemed that once women got to a "certain age," getaways were reserved for partners, spouses, and kids, not girlfriends (unless you counted weekend scrapbook parties, which I didn't). But for this trip, to my surprise and absolute delight, the timing for everyone was perfect, and a gang of seven gals had committed to go in November, just four months away.

As I strolled down the street to my minivan, with the midsummer sun warming my face, I felt exhilarated. Another twenty-four hours without kids still stretched before me. I couldn't remember the last time I'd had lunch or hung out with my girlfriends on a Sunday afternoon. For seven years, I'd spent virtually every weekend running around catering to my kids and their activities. And usually I'd done it alone, since Robert was often out of town.

I passed by patio cafes and noticed all the adults hanging out—talking, eating, people-watching. So *this* is what childless adults do with their time on weekends. I couldn't stop smiling. *I'm like you,* I called to them in my mind. *It's just for today, but look, I'm enjoying a nice Sunday afternoon down here too!* I even noticed a few men checking me out. I wondered if any men had looked at me these past years . . . Not that I'd been aware of. I'd always been too preoccupied, pushing a stroller, holding kids' hands, and getting from point A to point B without losing a child or my sanity.

As I climbed into my minivan and started it up, I remembered the new CDs Tory had gifted me at lunch. I loaded them into my player and Fergie's "Big Girls Don't Cry" began to play. I pulled out of the parking lot, speakers cranked up high. As I sang along and shoulder-shimmied in my seat, I realized other drivers and pedestrians were looking at my car. *That's right guys,* I thought with a smile. *That loud dance music you hear is coming from a MINIVAN.*

CHAPTER 6

STAY-AT-HOME MOM MEETS A DOM

I LOGGED ONTO THE DATING website with new resolve. I'd made a decision: to eliminate the over-thirty-five age restriction I'd imposed. Surely there was no harm in seeing what the younger men had to say.

Within two hours I was flipping through so much new mail, I couldn't keep track of which young man was which. I wondered: *Did younger men secretly fantasize about being with an older woman? Did they actually believe they would have anything in common with me, or were they strictly sexually curious?* I had heard the term "cougar" before, which in my book, I am *not*—I hate the word. And I had recently learned that "MILF" stood for Mother I'd Like to Fuck (how endearing). Is that how these younger men saw me? Should I be flattered or appalled?

Some of their emails were so blatantly immature, I laughed out loud: "Hey baby, how YOU doin'?" "You are so HOT!!!!" or "Holy MILF?!" Most of their profiles were clones: they liked to "hang with friends," "go to the gym," and they were looking for some "fun." Their photo galleries commonly showed them with a beer bottle in hand, standing in a lineup of intoxicated friends.

I enjoyed the attention though, and I wrote and chatted to a few. I had no intention of pursuing any of them seriously; this was just harmless play.

It was 1:00 AM. I was getting bored but not tired. My eyes kept returning to an advertisement in the corner of the screen. It boasted to be a site for millionaire men and gorgeous women— "Sugar Daddies" (cue eyes rolling), and "Sugar Babes" (good God!). On a whim, I clicked on the link.

Surprisingly, it didn't look too shoddy. In fact, the site itself was professionally presented and their mission statement, which focused on coupling attractive, educated, and like-minded men and women, actually made sense to me. Maybe it would weed out the riff-raff?

I was feeling feisty, so I signed up. I revised my current profile and uploaded it with a few of my best photos. They paled in comparison to other women's photos; many had professional modeling shots. But why not try it out? It could prove entertaining at the very least.

An hour later, my profile was approved and I was officially a new "Sugar Babe" (eyes still rolling). It was late and time for bed. Yawning, I went to click out of email when a "new mail" icon flashed on my screen. I quickly opened the message:

> I certainly enjoyed your profile. Please review mine and if it intrigues you, instead of making you run away screaming, please contact me . . .
> The Duke

The *Duke?* PU-leeze. I clicked on his profile:

> I'm a Dominant alpha male with two basic kinks (and a zillion small ones). First, I am very attracted to strong, confident, Dominant women—the "alpha females"—and I like them to be sexually submissive to me. I like a lioness that desires the intimate company of a lion.

The second thing is even kinkier. I like helping to create "monsters"—powerful, take-no-shit, demanding women who want to rule submissive or beta males for sport. I've been involved with a number of women whom I helped find and express their full alpha-femaleness through exerting their power over men . . . and I found it very satisfying.

So if you are a top-shelf alpha female not afraid of the work needed to be a woman like that, or the responsibilities in that (it's a sin for a nimrod male to take advantage of an alpha female), and you are looking for a partner/mentor to support you in pursuing your alpha dreams, then let me know. (If you are bi, that would also be very nice.)

Besides the company of confident, fun women, other interests include art, classic movies, and investing.

Wow. I reread his profile. *Wow again.*

I didn't really understand what he meant by Dominant/submissive. But for some reason, I was drawn to his words. He seemed confident and strong and, well . . . *experienced*. I wondered what it would be like to hang out with someone like him—inside and outside the bedroom.

Suddenly, my inner voice shrieked: *Are you crazy? He's probably some freak who's into leather and whips!* Visions of a skinhead wearing a studded collar and a sinister grin flashed through my mind.

"Oh relax," I grumbled and rolled my eyes. Seriously, if I took an objective, *nonhysterical* look at his profile, his writing suggested a man who was well educated and who possessed a strong respect for women. In fact, it sounded like he wanted to empower women.

My eyes moved to his photo at the side of the page. His head was cropped off, but I could tell that he was a large, heavily built man. My "headless" admirer stood with his hands on his waist, wearing jeans and a pastel green shirt with big white flowers on it. *Okay, obviously not the best dresser,* I grinned. *And those bright-white running shoes should only be worn at the gym.* Still, I felt intrigued. He had big hands, big arms, a thick waist; even his stance was strong, like a man who commanded attention.

I continued scouring his profile for other clues. It listed him as forty-eight years old; *hmmm . . . a bit out of my age bracket . . . Ah, he's six foot three*—I was right, he *is* a big man . . . Jeepers, he lives in New York—that's kind of far . . . His work is apparently "Internet-related," which is kind of cool, because my business (which I've neglected terribly) is e-based. His annual income? More than one million USD. His net worth? Five to ten million USD.

I'm certainly not at all what one would call a "gold digger." Money alone isn't enough to interest me; I see it as more of a bonus. In fact, this past summer during my serial dating rampage, I'd met *and* rejected a few millionaires.

But still, my imagination wandered. At this point in my life, I wanted to experience new things. And the idea of being treated like a queen by a successful, powerful man appealed to me. *Yes,* I grinned, *I could enjoy being swept away on a few exotic trips.* But more than that, I would enjoy having an intense mental connection with such a man. I envisioned myself waking up in a king-size bed in a penthouse somewhere, 600-thread-count Egyptian cotton caressing my skin, a sexy, ultra-intelligent man lying beside me. *Oh my god, could I get any more cliché!* I thought. But a woman's allowed to have her daydreams—stay-at-home moms too! So what if I wasn't a supermodel. I was smart enough and educated enough to keep any one of these guys on their toes, for a little while anyway.

I scoured his photograph one more time. This "Duke" guy could be a total cracker jack or an imposter. On the other hand, maybe he wasn't. Maybe he *was* authentic. A man of his thinking might make a good friend or mentor, maybe even a lover, though this Dominant/submissive stuff both scared and enticed me.

Since I was on a roll this weekend, why not see what was behind door number two?

So I wrote him back.

THE KIDS WERE in bed, fast asleep. Down in my office, I stared at the minute hand on my clock. After exchanging a few emails the past few days, I'd agreed to talk to The Duke by phone. Tonight. I was so nervous, I'd jotted down questions on a piece of paper. When the phone rang at precisely 9:00 PM, I knew it was him. But I let it ring four times to seem less eager.

"Is this Delaine?" asked a deep voice.

"Yes, it is. Hello Duke, how are you?" I asked, trying to sound calm and confidant.

"Very well. Let's begin by answering some of your questions, shall we?"

Shocked, I hid the paper behind my back. *Huh?*

"You said in your email you didn't understand what I meant by Dominant and submissive. So let's start there."

"Oh. Yes. Sounds good," I replied, whacking my palm against my temple. *God, I'm such an ass!*

Immediately he explained that he wasn't into whips and chains and sadomasochism *Phew.* His interest, he said, lay more on the "mental side" of domination, though at times, he might also include physical elements such as teasing and spanking. "Before we even went into the bedroom, I might grab you by the hair, look you straight in the eyes, and tell you that you are going to do everything I want," he said, his voice deep and matter-of-fact in my ear. "And you would submit to me . . . Because you *respected* me. And because you know I'm worthy."

"Being submissive to an alpha male does not make you a weakling or a doormat," he clarified. "Alpha females are very capable, confident, strong-minded women who normally have a dozen things on the go. But some part of them wants to relinquish control; they want a strong alpha man to take charge and challenge them, because with that comes an intensity and creative connection unlike anything they could experience in a regular or 'vanilla' relationship."

"There are many men out there pretending to be Dominants or alpha men," he went on. "But in actuality, they are 'beta men,' who are riddled with insecurities. They may appear successful and self-assured on the exterior, but underneath they are 'wannabes': Their identities are locked into their accomplishments and they live in constant fear of being exposed. I've sat in many meetings with these kinds of men before. They're easy to pick out. They're either pompous and arrogant or complete ass-suckers. It often comes out in how they talk about women: They put them down, treat them like objects. It's disgusting. I've had to sit there listening to them, all the while itching to punch them out."

"The worst thing that can happen to an alpha woman is be in a relationship with a beta man," he said with conviction. "He will bring her down, be jealous of her accomplishments, and consistently hold her back or sabotage her efforts, often unconsciously. This beta man doesn't deserve her—and he may or may not know it."

"A true alpha male," he continued, "is one whose confidence comes from within. There's no pretending, no need to be egotistical; he knows who he is. Often, these men are very successful and wealthy, but not always. Having money is certainly not proof alone of an alpha male," he warned. "There are lots of super rich trust-fund babies out there who are 'pathetic little boys with hard-ons.' Conversely, there are also many rich men out there who are so accustomed to getting what they want that they in turn feel a need to be submissive. They want to hand over control, be humiliated, beg for sex, or whatever their fetish may be, because some part of them doesn't want all that power."

As I listened to Duke talk, I paced the room, the phone pressed to my ear. My mind raced to process his ideas. Some seemed overly simplistic and superficial to me. But some were alluring, and I felt my body respond to them. My brain rushed to filter my own life through his looking glass: *Am I an alpha female?* I thought about all I manage and had managed for years as a full-time mother of three young kids; *pfft*, that was a CEO position if I'd ever seen one. I thought back to all the moms groups and meditation groups I had pioneered, how I'd worked full-time pre-kids, while also attending school and starting my own counseling practice. Even all the overseas travelling and moving I did in my twenties were indicative of a woman who was ferociously independent and bold. I'd just never felt comfortable with the label "Type A" or "alpha" personality. To me, being a leader meant being perceived as a bitch. I'd rather be well-liked, but seen as self-sufficient.

My thoughts shifted to Robert: *Is he an alpha male?* Without knowing it, I think I judged him to be one when I'd dated him. I thought he'd stood out as the alpha leader of his pack of friends. From the outside he was strong, rugged, handsome; he exuded what I deemed to be the quintessence of masculinity. His personality ranged from being confident and gregarious—the life of the party—to being quiet and private, a man of few words. But did he "know" himself? Was he self-aware and secure in who he was? Not at all. I'd mistaken his masculine bravado for alphaness. And consequently, I had put myself at risk, trying to forge a meaningful relationship with someone who was both afraid and intimidated by *my* power; all his bullying and put-downs were meant to "keep me in my place."

"So are you dating someone, Delaine?" the Duke was asking.

"Er—no," I said pulling my thoughts back to the present. "I dated a hockey player a while back. But his penis was really small and well, the sex was lame." *I can't believe I just said that to a man!*

Duke's response caught me off guard: "Being with a lame lover disrespects you, and I don't like anyone disrespecting you, even *you*. I'd like to take you over my lap and spank you right now for this. I'd spank you, then grab you by the hair and look in your eyes and tell you that from now on *you let no one disrespect you*. If it happens, you have to answer to *me*. I don't want you spreading your legs for 'lame,' *got it?*"

"I'm not making a habit of it!" I defended, wondering why I felt aroused by his verbal reprimands. "I've been out with a dozen men since him and I didn't see any of them beyond first date." I paused. "Actually, I *did* consider *one*, but at the end of our date, he grabbed me, kissed me, and soaked my face." I laughed.

"TWO things here," he stated. I gripped the phone, waiting. "FIRST, this is the kind of guy you should have slapped or painfully squeezed his nuts. I'd give you another spanking right now if I could. Nobody *takes* from you without your permission. Allowing this to happen was a 'bad Delaine' moment. Get this: You are nobody's doormat anymore. You got that?

"SECONDLY, regarding the other eleven men, you rejected them because they aren't good enough for you. That's good. No one should have a piece of you who doesn't deserve it. It's a sin. But the problem is, you're becoming more and more sexually frustrated in the interim. You aren't actually happy because your pussy isn't getting what it wants. There's a slut in you that is not being satisfied."

My mouth flew open in shock. *How dare he call me a slut!* "A slut," he explained, as if hearing my thoughts, "is a woman who likes to orgasm. Look it up. The current version. And you *do* like to orgasm. Don't you." It was a statement, not a question. Part of me wished I could slap him, yet another part roused in acknowledgement; no one had ever spoken to me like this before.

Then, for reasons unknown, I told him about my rendezvous with Yummy Stranger. He wasn't appalled or shocked like most men would be. Instead, he responded matter-of-factly: "You can choose to use boy toys as you please. You're allowed to have sex with whomever you choose. *But,* if you'd been smart, you'd have made him your ongoing submissive. What happens when next week you're going stir crazy for sex again? You should have told him as he left that you would call him again when you wanted him."

No way, I thought to myself. I really don't want to see Yummy Stranger again. That afternoon was a fantasy unto itself and was done. But he *was* right: What *do* I do next weekend when I'm raging for sex again? I'm in the same boat as before.

Duke continued, "You always have three choices available to you: dominate, submit, or reject. That's how relationships work. That's how the world works."

Is it really that cut and dry? I wondered. *Is this something men know about, but women don't?* I couldn't help but think of how easily I'd been walked on by Robert and Graham. Are men thinking in terms of power while women are buried up to their eyeballs in romance novels?

"Look Duke," I finally said, "I think that what I need to do is get more in touch with my masculine side. I'm very in tune with my feminine side, and I'm proud of that. But at this point, I don't think being more feminine will help me. I want to be more self-assured and aggressive at times. I want to take without apology when I'm rightfully entitled. I want to be mentally, emotionally tougher. I need the masculine."

"Your sexuality will translate into your day-to-day life," he told me. "There really is a domino effect. So much of the world is, at its core, about power, and sexual power is the rawest way to express that. Business is about dominance and submission, alpha and beta. Learn to appreciate your sexual power and the rest of the world comes in to better focus."

I was fascinated to have attracted a man like The Duke into my life. Why not some regular, simple, local guy? Out of all the millions of people on the Internet, why did I attract *him*?

I don't believe in coincidences; I believe there is a reason for everything that happens, and everyone we meet. Furthermore, I believe that "like energy" attracts "like energy," and that energy knows no time or space; that whether we are in the Arctic or Peru, we are like powerful radars, constantly emitting our mental and emotional signals, and attracting the perfect people and situations into our lives.

Perhaps Internet dating is the most brilliant example of that energy at work. We refer to cyberspace as being but an "electronic domain," but maybe it's more real and intuitive than we think.

I imagined emails—the thoughts and feelings of millions of people—zooming above the planet, searching, scanning, and connecting perfectly with those of others. I thought about all the different men I'd attracted thus far from cyberspace: hockey fighter Cal and all my serial dates. I then imagined my emails, my energy, traveling across Canada and the United States and locking onto The Duke's like an electromagnetic coupling.

Yes, attracting Duke was no accident. But I was kind of scared of him too. What if he really was a highly intelligent sociopath?

I laughed at myself: *He lives far away, Delaine. It was a harmless phone call.*

Besides, even if he is trying to brainwash me, I'm a smart lady. I'm wiser and more mistrustful than I've ever been in my life.

CHAPTER 7
RED LIGHT MEANS GO

MIDWEEK, HALI PHONED TO SAY she was going to check out a new lingerie shop that just opened, and would I like to join her? My knee-jerk response was to say no. I *should* be spending that time at home with my daughter and cleaning the house, as per usual. *Bah! Live a little, Delaine*, I suddenly thought. The floors could wait and Jenna could have a playdate at her friend's house.

An hour later, Hali and I met in front of Miss Chiff's Closet. I could tell by the mannequins in the window that this wasn't Victoria's Secret: On display were leather dresses and whips, a sexy maid costume, and high heels that even Barbie would gape at.

Problem was, the front doors were locked. The sign said it opened at 10:00 AM, and it was already ten after. Since Teah was asleep in her car seat and there was a coffee shop close by, we decided to grab a quick tea.

"So I'm a little surprised at this," I said, after we'd settled in at a table with steaming mugs. "What made you want to check this place out?"

Hali smiled without an ounce of timidity, and shrugged. "I just checked out their website and it seemed very empowering to women, like it caters to the woman's imagination and pleasure, not just the guy's. And the lingerie is higher-end, too." Hali paused to take a sip of her tea, while I casually eyeballed the café to see if anyone might be listening in; the only other patron, a woman in a business suit and glasses, appeared fully engrossed in her book. I leaned over the table eagerly, prodding her. "Well what else?"

She smiled and leaned in to, dropping her voice a bit. "They also offer stripping classes for women—not professional stripping classes, just techniques on how to strip for your man," she said, adding with a mischievous grin, "I might take a class."

I smiled back. I was half in awe of this new side of her. All these years, I'd viewed her as reserved, very prim and proper. She'd always kept her hair cut short, and her dress style was conservative but elegant, mainly because of her male-dominated career in financial planning. I'd always felt like a bit of a flower child next to her. Certainly, I could dress up when called for, but day in, day out, I was a faded blue jeans, T-shirt, and handmade jewelry kind of girl. Side by side, we were like Sheryl Crow and the Prime Minister's wife.

Now as I looked at her across the table, with her sexy, longer hairstyle and more fashionable attire, I realized her blossoming sexuality was transforming her from the inside out. Even though her life was in chaos, I could sense a new power about her.

"Are you planning to strip for Josh?" I asked.

"No!" she replied firmly. "There's no doubt that he helps me feel good about my body. But this is more about *my* sexuality. I want to explore it. Maybe it's because I'm approaching forty, or maybe it's because of what I've been through." She sat back and took another sip of tea. "I know the sex is exciting right now because it's with someone new. But I really think it's more than that. I'm trying new things in bed, I'm becoming less inhibited, I want to learn how to be a better lover—not for them, but for me."

She leaned forward and lowered her voice even more. "All these years, I've never enjoyed giving blow jobs—not because I hated it, but because I didn't think I was any good at it. I was talking to Patty the other day, and she said she found a video online that gives step-by-step instructions on how to give *the* best blow job. She said it was amazing and even she had being doing things wrong."

"So what are these steps?" I asked. Surely I had room for improvement, too.

Suddenly, for a flash of second, I thought of being down on my knees in front of Robert. Planning my day. Willing him to hurry up with my thoughts and hands. What if that scenario presented itself in a future relationship? Once the newness wore off, would I end up in the exact same position emotionally as I was before?

I shook off the thoughts and tuned in closely as Hali began discreetly explaining *and* demonstrating blow job highlights. I smiled and began taking mental notes. I suddenly felt a rush of immense gratitude for the women in my life—our openness and honesty with each other was a source of true personal empower-ment. I wondered if my mother had ever talked with her girlfriends like this when she was younger—especially with a newborn baby lying in a car seat beside their table.

JUST AFTER ELEVEN o'clock, Hali and I were back at Miss Chiff's Closet, browsing through the clothes with grins plastered across our faces: policewoman, sexy nurse, latex dominatrix, full body fishnets . . . Bet they did great business here on Halloween. It was hard to imagine myself wearing it any other time of year.

"Hey Hali, is there something specific you're looking for?"

"Oh, I don't know. Something I feel good in. Something sexy. Something *slutty,* " she added, laughing.

"Well, you've certainly come to the right place," I said dryly, holding up a black, sleeveless minidress that had large holes cut down the front. "How about something like *this?*"

Hali laughed. "Jesus, is that a dress? It looks small enough to fit your daughter!" She suddenly looked inspired. "Hey! Why don't *you* try it on?"

I frowned. "Nah—I wasn't planning to shop for me."

"Oh, c'mon, try it on," she begged, giving me a faux sad face. "You have the body for it."

Hmmm. Maybe I would, I thought. *Just for fun.* I'd never actually wear something like this. But, there again . . . that was the knee-jerk reaction of practical Delaine, down-to-earth mother of three *very* small children. It felt frivolous and indulgent. *Oh screw it! Just cause I'm a mom doesn't mean I have to be milquetoast. I can be sensuous and adventurous, if I want to be!* Especially with a man like The Duke. The sudden thought of him sent a little zing of pleasure through my body. Maybe he'd *make* me wear something decadent. Suddenly, I felt more motivated. It would be nice to have something naughty tucked away for "special occasions."

Over the next hour, we were like giddy schoolgirls on back-to-school shopping day, scampering back and forth a dozen times from the changing room to the clothing racks. I was intoxicated with the fun and the sense of liberation it engendered, because with each garment I tried on, my imagination took flight. Not just with visions of me wearing it, but with how that woman might feel about herself as she wore it and who she might grow into one day. The possibilities were endless; this wasn't about "dressing" my skin, but exploring what and who lay within me. Delaine the Sexually-Numb Wife wouldn't have been caught dead in this store; God, why give her husband more incentive? Delaine the Love-Sick Mistress wouldn't have lurked here either, for no other reason than because her lover Graham thought lingerie was "slutty." But Delaine the Soon-to-be Divorcee had no man in the wings; no need to please or impress. The only reason she was in this store was because she wanted to be. It was her choice. And she liked it. Being in a shop that breathed with sexual mischief reconnected her with the feelings of passion and adventure she'd felt in her twenties. At the same time, it felt like a whole new land of discovery, for she was reentering this world at a different age and different stage of her life.

One hour later, I left the store carrying the inconspicuous "black bag." I'd bought a glamorous pink corset, thigh-high fishnet stockings, and two very skimpy, "bedroom only" dresses. Grinning, I thought of Hali, who was last seen in the store feeding her daughter a bottle in a black latex minidress and high-heeled boots. *Dominatrix Momma.*

As I walked toward my car in the midday sunshine, I laughed to myself.

When am I ever going to wear this stuff?

As it turned out, just two days later.

HALI PHONED ME Friday morning, excited. "So I took the stripping class last night."

Why was I not surprised? "How was it?"

"Great," she said, dismissively. Apparently, she had more important news to share.

"After everyone left, I was there with just the teacher. And all night long I had been wondering, what the heck *is* this place? It almost looked like a condo, but there were high tables and stools, like in a bar, and a dance floor with a pole—which we learned to work, by the way. The room actually looked quite elegant. But I didn't understand why a place like this was located way out in an industrial area. It was in a warehouse building, and there were no signs on the outside door.

"I kept asking my teacher, 'Is this someone's condo? Does someone live here?' But she kept avoiding my questions. Eventually, she gave in: 'Actually, it's a *sex club.*'"

"Wow. *Really?*" I asked, incredulous. "I've heard of them before, but I didn't know there was one in Calgary."

I sat there on the phone, waiting for Hali to express her disgust. I assumed these places attracted desperate, sleazy men, and that did *not* interest me. But instead, she said, "I want to go."

"WHAT? *What!* Are you out of your flippin' mind?"

"No, I'm not," she said laughing. "I really want to go. *Tonight.* They're having a party and I want to go. And I want you to come with me."

I had to laugh too. "Hali, you're crazy."

"We don't have to *do* anything. We can just go and check it out. I looked at the club's website and talked to the woman in charge. It's not at all what you think. You have to be screened to get in. No single men are allowed; only single women and couples. They have over four hundred members. Tonight, the theme is 'Wear What You Dare.'"

"Ohhhh, Hali," I said, shaking my head. "Wear What You *Dare?*"

"Yes. A perfect opportunity to wear your new pink corset."

"Yeah, right."

"The owner assured me it is *not* sleazy at all. She said their clientele are mainly professionals, the kind you'd see downtown in a suit on a Friday afternoon. You would never know they go to a sex club. She also said that in this club, a woman's choice is always put first—no means no, and it must be respected at all times. We are not obligated to do anything. We can just watch if we want."

"Soooo . . . how does a first-time visit work then?"

"Well, first you have to fill out a form on their website . . ."

As Hali went over the registration how-to's, I sat on the line, trying to swallow Hali's proposition. I exhaled loudly; so many questions—*ethical* questions: Even if we didn't participate in any sexual goings on, could we be considered indecent or corrupt just for visiting such a place? What if something actually happened? What if we *liked* it? What if we ran into someone we knew? What if we bumped into someone from the sex club somewhere else in the future?

"Okay, okay," I sighed. "What's the name of the website?" I was totally fascinated but a little disgusted, too. Warning bells rang in my head like a truck in reverse: Stay clear! Back up! Don't go this way!

Why do I consider this so lurid? I wondered. *What was wrong with consenting adults mingling in this way? Who was I to judge the spectrum of sexual expression? Is there even a barometer?* In my mind's eye, I saw myself standing alone in a spotlight. A game show host is whispering to a hushed audience. "Will she take the challenge folks? THAT is the million-dollar question. Or will she turn her back and stick with her cloistered stay-at-home mom existence?

Screw it!

I promised to fill out and submit the application. "I'll ask my sitter if she's free after the kids are in bed tonight."

"Thanks, Delaine!" said Hali, clearly elated. "I don't know why I'm so curious about this, but I really want to see what it is. And I won't do it unless *you* come. I can't ask anyone else but you."

I hung up the phone and immediately logged onto the club's website. I browsed around attentively, searching suspiciously for sleaze or any red flags. Instead, it reiterated a lot of what Hali had told me, highlighting their many rules, requirements, and policies. The site itself was very tasteful and professionally presented. I navigated to the application page and ten minutes later pressed "send."

Then I walked over to my children's school and joined the other moms who were picking up their kids for lunch.

HALI AND I agreed to meet at the Big Town shopping mall parking lot and drive to the club together. I'd squeezed into my pink corset, feeling sexy but exposed. *How could I leave the house in this?*

I thought. Hali planned to deck herself out in a latex dress, with a cardigan over the top, just in case.

Driving in my minivan, with Shakira belting out "Hips Don't Lie," I felt weirdly *free*. I was up for the adventure, whatever it would be. I turned the music up, grooving in my seat and singing along. My minivan suddenly felt more like a dance club on wheels than a mommy-mobile, with its empty car seats and stale Cheerios. After years of tolerating toddler and kids' tunes to make car rides bearable, I had forgotten just how much I enjoyed dance music. How many renditions of "The Wheels on the Bus" had I endured? I'd listen to anything in lieu of sitting in rush-hour traffic with three screaming toddlers in the car. Oh, the number of red lights I had willed to turn to green . . .

I looked out the window as I sped through the night, and the glimmering lights of the downtown core winked back at me, inviting me to discover its hidden secrets.

HALI'S CAR SAT idling in the middle of the mall parking lot. I pulled up alongside her and got out—gingerly. *Damn corset.*

I opened her passenger door and sat down—*gingerly*. Hali was putting on lipstick in her rearview mirror. "Okay," I said, "So how are you doing?"

"I'm good," she said, automatically. Then she looked at me. "But I'm nervous. Are you?"

"Yes!" I laughed. "This is crazy. Absolutely *freaking crazy*. But, whatever." I leaned back in the chair. "Let's do it."

The club was located in the back of a long, monochrome industrial building. Except for the club's unmarked black doors, this side of the building was as dull as the front. It felt like gangster territory, and behind these closed doors I imagined smoky poker rooms and car thieves reassembling stolen parts. Hali and I were completely silent.

"That's it there," she half-whispered, "The one with the small red light out front." She parked a few doors down, but kept the car running.

"It's kind of funny that it has a red light," I said lightly. "It's like we're going into the red-light district."

"You sure you want to do this?" asked Hali, nervously rubbing her hands.

"ME? *You're* the one who wanted to come! And now, *yes*, I want to check it out. We didn't come here to just sit in a parking lot. It's right there, we look great, so let's go—before I lose my courage." I opened the door. "Worst-case scenario, we stay for ten minutes then leave."

"Okay."

My heart beat faster as we approached the entrance. I lifted my chin, thrust my shoulders back, and swung open that door like I owned the place.

We stepped into a dimly lit entryway. Further passage was blocked by another closed door, beyond which I could hear dance music. To our left, a man and woman sat behind what appeared to be a coat check. *Phew, they're both dressed.*

"Hi," the woman said loudly. "Can I help you?" Not friendly, but guarded. *She's a watchdog.*

"Hi, my name is Hali. I spoke with the owner earlier today, and my friend, Delaine, and I are visiting for the first time tonight."

The man behind the desk was looking at me as Hali talked. He was slim and short—maybe five foot seven—and had a goatee. I half-smiled at him and tried not to fidget. His appraising look made me feel even more self-conscious than I already did. Guard Woman pulled out a sign-in sheet and pointed. "I need you to write your name *here* and sign *here*. I also need to see your driver's licenses."

Yes Ma'am! I quickly jumped to do her bidding.

"And *I'll* take your jackets," said the man with the goatee, his voice rich, creamy . . . like butter. I felt naked as I shrugged it off my bare shoulders into his hands.

He can't see anything, I reminded myself. *Just relax!*

But he knows you're sexually curious! That's why you're here! trilled a panicked voice in response.

Front door admin complete, Goatee Man opened the inside door. "Welcome ladies," he said with a brush of his arm, and we stepped into a large room. It was much like Hali had described: a bit like a condo, but in lieu of living room furniture, bar tables and stools were spread across the hardwood floors. About fifteen people were scattered around the dimly lit room, but I didn't dare look at anyone directly. Instead, I looked around them and above them, at sensual red-wine walls and dark wooden tabletops. The overall feel was warm. Mysterious. *Sexual.*

"I see you brought some alcohol," Goatee Man said. I looked down—yes, I had forgotten. Knowing the club wasn't licensed, I had grabbed a half-bottle of white wine out of my fridge on my way out the door.

Goatee Man walked over to a bar and poured our wine into glasses for us. "Allow me to show you around," he offered graciously. "And feel free to ask any questions you may have as we go along." Hali and I quickly sipped our wine.

As Goatee Man went over the club's rules, I stood close to Hali, only half listening. I was dying of self-consciousness. *Were people sizing me up as new meat?*

". . . and toward the end of the night, you'll see that a lot of people leave this area and go upstairs," I heard him say.

There's an upstairs? Hali and I followed him back toward the entrance and up a set of stairs. No one else was up there. Away from the scrutiny of others, I calmed down somewhat. Goatee Man led us to an area on the right that held the same furnishings as any comfortable living room: couches, side tables, coffee table, artwork on the wall; there was even a TV in the corner, which was on. But it wasn't a sitcom playing, it was porn. And the paintings were erotic as well. Goatee Man continued, in a very matter-of-fact tone: "You'll find on the side tables anything you might need—condoms, towels, wet naps . . ."

"You mean people will actually come up here to have *sex?*" I blurted.

"Yes." He guided us to another room; this one had jail bars as a door. "If you want some privacy, feel free to come in here." I peeked inside. Two fully made-up queen-size beds lay side by side against chocolate-colored walls. Between them hung a painting of an open vagina. I noted that the wine-red bed pillow matched the labia in the artwork. *Whoa. They don't miss anything.*

"And over here—" he led us across a bridge illuminated by tiny white floor lights, ". . . again, we have couches set up with all the amenities you might need. This room is often used for group activities. And way over there—" he pointed to the far corner, ". . . we have a Saint Andrew's cross and other scene paraphernalia. That section is popular on Saturday nights, which is our Fantasy Night for dominants and submissives. But all members are welcome to use it any night they wish," he added, smiling politely.

We made our way back to the top of the stairs. Goatee Man wrapped up: "You don't have to participate in anything up here. You can simply watch if you like. Some of our members are exhibitionists and love an audience," he added, smiling. "While others are into voyeurism. But, if someone asks you *not* to watch, you are expected to respect her wishes. I can't say strongly enough, no means no here. Women's choice comes first and must be obeyed at all times. You will see us walking around, monitoring the goings-on of the night to ensure that all our members are safe and happy."

I was taken aback but also reassured by his businesslike manner, as if he was showing us around a resort hotel. Hali and I made our way back downstairs and found a table near the back of the room by the dance floor. I was starting to feel a little buzz from the wine and was finally relaxing. I scanned the room quickly, then again, more slowly. Everyone was busy doing his or her own thing: socializing, laughing, sometimes in small groups, some just in pairs. I noticed that most of the men were fully dressed in business-casual attire. But a number of women were wearing more daring outfits, and they came in various shapes and sizes.

I stared inconspicuously at two older women at a table close by. One appeared to be around fifty and wore a skimpy, black bedroom dress like the one I bought at Miss Chiff's Closet (the one full of holes). Her companion was a beautiful heavy-set woman, who also revealed skin and curves with no apparent concern. They both seemed so relaxed and comfortable—here *and* in their bodies. I observed their husbands, who both looked like businessmen: One bald, one bulging at the belt, they were absorbed in conversation.

At the back of the room, Hali and I quietly shared our observations. We noted that the youngest group of people in the room was in our age bracket. They were socializing as if at a pub. Two other couples in their forties were dancing and chatting on the dance floor; one woman looked like Sally Homemaker in her grey and pink-checkered vest.

A couple of men and women approached us for casual conversation. But we both quickly expressed that it was our first time here. I think we scared them off.

"Oh my God," I heard Hali murmur.

"What?"

"Don't look now, but you know those older women a few tables over? I think they just switched husbands." I casually looked over and . . . yup, yes-sir, no-doubt-about-it-folks—a switchover had transpired. Not only were the husbands openly touching the other's wife, one woman was rubbing the other woman, too.

I didn't want to stare but I couldn't help it. Obviously they weren't uncomfortable exhibiting, so why should I be shy about watching?

My body and brain were noticeably warm and fuzzy from the wine. The music was getting louder. And the songs being played were current, sexy; perfect for dancing and grinding. Sally Homemaker paraded back onto the dance floor with her husband and another man in tow, and it wasn't long before she was being grilled, fried, and sandwiched.

"Look," whispered Hali. "They're going upstairs." The two older couples had disappeared as a group up the stairs. Hali couldn't resist adding commentary: "Going upstairs for some action, folks."

I reached for my wine glass to help me chase down what I was witnessing. But dammit, it was empty! I wished I'd brought more.

Meanwhile, over at the pub-like gathering of younger adults, one of the women had taken off her jacket, showing off her assets. Her tall, slim frame was covered only by a lacy G-string and black leather chaps. The cutest man over there (Hali and I had agreed) was now squeezing and necking a luscious-looking black woman with a long mane of hair.

Suddenly, movement above me caught my eye. I looked up and realized that I could clearly view the upper floor. And directly facing me was the Saint Andrew's cross. Black Minidress Woman was being tied onto it by her bald husband. The other woman was across from her, but I couldn't see her. I *could*, however, see the top of her husband's head; I think he was strapping her into something, too.

Once Minidress Woman was bound to the cross, her husband lifted her skirt, exposing her spread-eagled nakedness for all to see. He stood in front of her, kissing her, his hand visibly playing elsewhere. She smiled and talked. Sometimes she tilted her head back against the cross, obviously enjoying the pleasure she received. I pulled my eyes away, wishing even harder that I'd brought more wine.

I looked up again. A man was still in front of her but . . . hold on, people. It was now the other woman's husband. They were switching back and forth!

"Wow, Hali," I exhaled heavily. "This is turning me on."

"Yeah, it's super sexually charged," replied Hali, who'd been observing the upstairs' events too. "I'm glad I had sex three times last night," she said with a sly grin.

"You *did*? But I thought you went to the stripping class!"

"And afterward, Josh came over."

"Well I've had sex maybe six times in a flippin' year and this is really getting to me!"

"Do you want to go upstairs and watch?" Hali half-teased half-dared.

"*God* no! No *way!* I don't want to participate in anything. Watching from here is more than enough."

But soon, the electricity in the room began to frustrate me. "Hali, I've probably had the least amount of sex out of every person in this entire room and I'm sitting here watching everybody *else* get some," I said, exasperated. "I'm ready to go when you are."

It wasn't yet midnight as Hali drove me back to my car. But I felt like I'd just spent days in the Twilight Zone. "Wow," I exhaled. "That was something else."

"Yeah. It was *intense.* The entire place breathed with sex."

"So, are you glad you went?"

"For sure," she said. "It was great to experience it. But I wouldn't buy a membership," she added, emphatic. "I doubt I'll ever go back, though who knows with me these days. What about you?"

I thought for a minute, eyebrows knit. My feelings weren't totally black and white. "Well, it definitely pushed me out of my comfort zone. Right now I really want to have sex, so it obviously worked for me on some level! The problem is, I've got zilcho in the playmate department and I don't think I could have simply hooked up with a stranger there tonight—and in front of all those people—so I'm not sure what that means."

"Would you go back again?"

I thought again for a moment. "No, I don't think so. A part of me is a bit curious about their Fantasy Night, the whole dominant/submissive thing. But I doubt I'll follow up. When it comes right down to it, I think it was neat to experience it, but it's not me."

"See? I think that's what's so cool about this, Delaine: We're growing, changing, trying new things; yet when it comes right down to it, whether we'd decided to go upstairs or not, we're capable of making choices that work for us. Other people would probably judge us just because we set foot in a sex club. But *we* know we can step outside our box and still be true to ourselves."

Hali pulled up beside my parked minivan, and we continued talking. The night didn't just test our comfort zone, it galvanized thought. We were both bursting to share our personal insight about our sexuality. "The fact that people knew, beyond a doubt, that I was there because I was sexually curious made me really uncomfortable," I admitted. "When I go to a bar, I can sit in the corner, play coy, and pretend like I'm not there to pick up. But at this place, as soon as we walked through the doors, I couldn't hide: I was willingly entering a sex club, so I was openly admitting that I was there because of the sex. That was an uncomfortable feeling for me to sit in."

"But I can see how that's empowering too," said Hali. "You're forced to acknowledge and sit tall in your own sexuality. I think as women we're taught to deny and suppress our sexuality from the time we're teenagers. We're taught that good girls don't say or act a certain way. But the bottom line is, as grown women we are entitled to use and enjoy our bodies however we please. We are sexual beings and no one should be allowed to make those decisions for us. Our bodies belong to *us*."

"I totally agree, but I don't know about the swinging thing." I raked my hand through my hair. "Watching those couples switch partners brought up mixed feelings for me."

"I know it wouldn't work for me," Hali said emphatically.

"But since both of us were cheated on and millions of others are cheating as we speak, doesn't it make you question if people are meant to be monogamous?" I pushed. "Or if maybe we overassign meaning to sex? If the people we saw tonight truly believe that sex can be but a pleasurable act and not feel the possessiveness and jealousy the rest of us do, maybe their chances of staying together are greater than ours. Because they wouldn't need to lie and deceive each other, like our husbands did to us. And wasn't it the deception that really killed our marriages?"

"So, are you saying that if Robert had approached you while you were pregnant and said, 'Look, I know you're not feeling horny these days but I am. So do you mind if I fuck someone else while you throw up?'—THAT would have made it easier?"

I laughed. "No! Though a part of me would've been relieved to have him stop bugging me for sex. Seriously though, I think it's impossible for us to imagine what it 'could' be like, Hali, when our current rigid beliefs around sex have been force-fed to us since we were young. They're so deeply ingrained in us that we can't even begin to shift out our lenses. Hell, we don't even know that we may want to *change* our lenses or that we're even wearing them." I paused, as that thought sat with me.

Hali suddenly pulled out her cell phone. "Josh just texted me!" she announced merrily. "I'm going to tell him to meet me."

"Well, you're certainly dressed for him," I said wryly, as I reached for the door. "Thanks for the most *memorable* evening, Miss Hali."

EVEN THOUGH IT was one in the morning, I went straight to my computer and logged onto the dating site. I didn't even bother to change or take off my high-heeled boots. As I sorted through my inbox, I clicked directly on the senders' profiles instead of opening their emails to see if they were good-looking. And the verdicts were: *No. No. Yuck, no. Oh look, it's Don.*

Don was one of the twelve men I met in person a couple of months ago. I actually found him very attractive; he was like a short Val Kilmer, but he had "player" written all over him; a bedpost notcher mixed in with a bit of gooey slime. Since our date, he'd continued to pursue me via email, sexual and flirtatious messages that always made me smile. This one read:

> Mmmmm, I wish we were together tonight. While you sat drinking your wine, I would start at your feet, gently kissing them, rubbing them. I'd slowly make my way up to your knees . . . thighs . . . You'd tilt your head back, trying not to spill your wine while I removed your panties . . . all the while touching you . . . licking you . . .

Yeah Don. I would actually enjoy you tonight, I thought with a sigh. But no. He was just too gooey.

Back to my inbox. Where was I? Oh, there. Next profile: *No . . . no . . . eww, creepy . . . hmmmm, maybe.* This guy was pretty cute; same age as me, too. Kind of looked like a high school quarterback: short thick hair, huge white smile . . . Wow. In his second photo, he was driving a quad with his shirt off—*very* nice chest. And in this last photo he was hugging a dog, a golden retriever.

I opened his message:

> Hi there beautiful. How's your night going? –Chad

Well, dear Chad, I mock replied in my head. *I just got back from a sex club and I'm sitting here in a corset and stockings.* Chuckling, I fired him a platonic reply.

I clicked on my own profile and examined my photos. They showed me in a range of attire: blue jeans, camouflage pants, a pretty dress, and an elegant pantsuit. Maybe I should spice up my collection a bit, I thought. It wouldn't hurt to throw in a sexier shot.

I turned on my webcam and fiddled with it till I figured out how to snap a picture. My photo shoot began.

Fifteen minutes later, I was viewing my self-taken photos with a huge smirk on my face. With no audience, I'd played up to the camera in a variety of poses: Good Girl casually lounging in a corset, Wild-Haired Vixen leaning over showing cleavage, Naughty Girl pulling her hair with a telltale smile. I laughed out loud as I perused them. Some were truly hilarious, and I looked like a total ass. But a couple of them were pretty good. I decided to add them to my profile gallery, even if just for the night.

Soon after, I was cozied up in bed, clean-faced and wearing my Super Girl pajamas. I wondered if I'd regret uploading those photos in the morning. But why should I hide the fact that I'm a sexual, desirable woman?

I thought back to what I witnessed at the sex club, particularly the older woman who was last seen strapped to the St. Andrew's cross. She hadn't the youthfulness or ideal body our society worships, yet she wore her skin with astounding confidence. She'd walked across the room like she owned the place. And she had commanded her sexual wants and desires with no apology. Maybe she understood something most people never have the guts to even daydream about.

I wondered what kind of work she did during the day . . . *I bet she works in an office,* I thought. I imagined that when she talked to colleagues, her voice was clear, her laugh unstifled. She was good at her job—intelligent, self assured, and capable. It just made sense to me that her confident sexuality would ripple into all areas of her life, like what The Duke had said. These were qualities I aspired to own and radiate, too. But *without* having to join a sex club.

CHAPTER 8
CHAMBER OF SELF-DOUBT

IT WAS THE BEGINNING OF a new school year, a time of firsts, new schedules, and fresh photos for the album. I shared my daughter's nervousness at attending her first day of preschool. As I packed her snack, I watched her out of the corner of my eye—her fingers twisting through her long dark hair, her bowl of Shreddies practically untouched. I tried to reassure her with my own stories from preschool: "And you're going to *color* and *paint* and *make crafts*. And oh, you're going to meet so many new friends!" Her doe eyes weren't convinced. Her fingers kept winding . . . coiling. *Please make this a wonderful day for my baby,* I silently prayed.

And when my eldest boys, now entering kindergarten and second grade, entered the kitchen fully dressed in their uniforms, I actually took a step back—they looked so grown up. "You're both so handsome!" I exclaimed as I leaned in to straighten ties and smooth collars. Besides their matching uniforms, my boys looked nothing alike—one extra tall with shaved blond hair, the other red- and curly-haired, with a smile that reeked of monkey business. Side by side they stood tall, little chests puffed out with pride. My little men . . . going out into the world.

I joined the other moms in the schoolyard and watched, in a daze, as my children waved and disappeared through the backdoors. *Time moves forward,* whispered the large oak trees surrounding the school.

Even though today was an important and somewhat emotional day, the degree of my attention felt forced—my ability to fully *feel* was forced. There was a time when such a day would have fulfilled me in every possible way; my kids' big day would have been *my* big day, too. But instead, it made me aware of that still-broken part of me: I start to feel an emotion—*any* kind of emotion—and then *smack*. I hit a wall of numbness. Or was it restlessness?

I tried not to beat myself up for my feelings. But my mother guilt kept hounding me. Because even though my kids were thriving and I'd shielded them from my divorce, even though I was back to devoting 95 percent of my time to them, my heart wasn't fully into my mommy job anymore. And it killed me—I'd always taken that job *very* seriously. Maybe even too seriously. Perhaps to the point where it, and my role as wife, defined who I was. Maybe that was where my identity crisis originated; maybe I'd begun losing who I was long before the men I loved ripped out my heart.

I'd always wondered if my leaving the work force was a smart choice. Not for the sake of my kids, but for ME. Because as much as I loved being a mom, as much as I recognized how it challenged me to grow as a woman and human being, I was always aware that it came with sizable price tags: my autonomy and financial independence. Oh, but sometimes I longed to engage in stimulating adult conversation, or collaborate on an exciting, important project of some kind! Better still to have had my hand shaken, respect earned, for a job well done. Sometimes, when I was overtired and besieged by the kids' tantrums and whining and crying, I not only thought, "God, I SUCK at being a mom" but "Did I *really* go to university for six years to do THIS?"

But I'd always shook such thoughts off, reminding myself that any job, be it at home or otherwise, would entail periods of feeling overwhelmed and dissatisfied. No—I promised myself I would *never* view my homemaker's role as a "sacrifice." To do so would negate the blessings and joys of what it offered me. Staying at home had been a *choice*, as are most things in life. And in turn I'd chosen to smile, accept it, and *embrace* it; no regrets.

When you cut right down to the core of what moms do, part-time or full-time, it's one thing: GIVE. You give of your soul, you give of your heart, you give of your breasts, your hands, your patience, your time, your love . . . And no matter how much you give, the job requires more, today, tomorrow, and every day after that. And that's what I'd done: give, love, and take care of everyone else, all day, all night, around the clock. Even when I was empty, exhausted, overwhelmed, *done,* I would dig deeper, shave off more of myself, and find "it," whatever "it" was that they needed, so that they would smile, calm down, hug me, get dressed, fall asleep, *stay* asleep. Giving and giving, always on alert, always anticipating their calls, cries, wants, fights, falls, pains. In my quest to be the ultimate supplier of love, patience, and energy, in the end, I had no reserves left for myself. I'd given *me* away. I hadn't known where to draw lines—or even to draw lines to begin with. I hadn't known to differentiate the wants and needs of them from *me.* Nor had I separated those of *Robert* from me. He blurred into the frenzied memory of my homemaker's life as a vision of one more hand reaching out, wanting something, *demanding* something. And I'd turn to him and smile . . . lie back and spread my legs . . . merging my self into his need, too.

Regardless of when or how I'd lost myself, I was angry that I was making my crisis all about me and what *I* was going through; three children's lives were also at stake. As a parent, you can't just suddenly go on sabbatical when life hits you between the eyes. Kids need their mom every day, ready or not. They *should* be able to rely on their mom. But what do you do when you *know* that, but you can't "will" your bashed-up heart to participate? How do you suddenly balance meeting all their many needs against the urgent demands of your own?

Fear descended upon me: *What if I feel this way forever? What if my kids are perceiving the change in my interest level and it causes some psychological breakdown later on in life?* I imagined my eldest son lying on some psychiatrist's couch, saying, "Well doc, I'd have to say that the turning point in my life was when my *mom* . . ."

I just wished I could accelerate my learning; hurry up and understand myself so I could get the hell out of this place. I understood that I wasn't supposed to be with Robert or Graham. I understood that there was a different plan for me. So when was the universe going to chuck me a fucking bone? (*Anybody up there listening?*) There again, maybe I deserved this. Maybe I was dealing with bad karma and this was my punishment for having had an affair. *(Spit)*

Anger. Self-pity. Despair. Then more anger, more self-pity, more hopelessness. The merry-go-round of emotions went round and round, mesmerizing me, seducing me into these dark aspects of myself—and I surrendered. Underneath it all, I desperately wanted someone to grab hold of my hand tightly and lead me in the right direction. Instead, all I had was me—broken, lost me, who right now believed that her recent choices were not only questionable, but maybe even unethical. If I was working on my business, which I'd hardly touched, or going back to school, maybe I'd have had more faith in my decision-making abilities; my *character*. Instead, I was dating up a storm, fantasizing about some dominant in New York City, and exploring sex clubs.

Still, it somehow felt right. A voice in my head kept telling me that this time of exploration was not only due me, it was necessary. *You have been through hell*, it whispered softly. *Now is your time to heal and grow.*

But *was* I growing? Or was I wasting precious time seeking thrills and acting out?

I couldn't even blame my feelings or behavior on Graham anymore. I'd hardly even thought of him over the past month. But I felt like a big black scab was holding my heart together—one wrong move and I'd find myself back at the entrance of the wilderness. I'd definitely made progress through the wilds: In my mind's eye, I no longer saw me stumbling along aimlessly with the burden of my grief on my back. The terrain before me was less rocky, and I was definitely walking taller. But my body felt restless . . . edgy.

Wherever this path was headed, I hadn't the resolve to change what I was doing. I was just following the path of least resistance, hoping for the best—or at least that it wouldn't get me into too much trouble. I knew I had about three years to get my career and financial future in order; that's what the latest draft of my separation agreement said, anyway. So instead of panicking over my timeline, I reminded myself that a lot could happen in three years. I *would* get my life organized again. I may not have charted a firm course yet, but with every small choice, every small task I completed every day, I was moving forward. I could beg and stomp my feet and cry as much as I wanted, but the bottom line was that I couldn't rush my evolution; the universe would send me a sign when I was ready.

My FASCINATION WITH The Duke was building—but so were my paranoia and fear around him. What if he'd made his Internet millions in the pornography business? Or maybe the Internet gig was a cover; maybe in real life he was a drug lord or operated a chain of strip joints. Worse still, maybe he was a pimp! Immediately, I sent him an email expressing my suspicions: What, did he think me just some naïve stay-at-home mom? *I'll show him who's "alpha"!* I thought determinedly.

But Shane was thoroughly amused, replying that I had a "twisted and wild imagination." Later that day, he then phoned to reassure me that his business dealings were aboveboard and honorable.

"Then why won't you tell me who you are?" I demanded. "And why won't you send me a photo of your face?"

"My *name* is Shane," he replied. "My *identity* is a whole other issue. Since you and I aren't taking any steps to meet at this point, I don't think it's necessary to disclose. Why do you need a photo anyway? To find out if you're attracted to me? *You already are.*"

I didn't want to admit it . . . but he was right. His mind had me hooked. I knew he was withholding his personal information to get a rise out of me *and* to establish his "dominant" status. If I wanted to keep talking to him—and I did—then I'd have to let it go.

No, I wasn't considering him as boyfriend material, though the role of kinky, out-of-town lover had crossed my mind. If anything, Shane was becoming like a "freaky life" coach, one whose mission was to train me to master myself through my sexuality.

His views and outlook on the world both repulsed and intrigued me. Power/sex/life—I'd never perceived the world through that triangle before. And though I didn't always agree with his opinions, I liked that he made me *think*; he made me *question.* Because looking around at my shambled life, I couldn't help but wonder, what didn't I "get"? Was I too naïve about love and relationships? Was I too heart-centered? Was I taught to believe in something(s) that doesn't even exist? After all, I'd followed all of society's well-mapped-out "rules": I got married, had kids, loved, trusted, sacrificed, worked hard, and wholeheartedly believed in both Robert and Graham. How might I prevent disaster from happening again? I was looking for answers, missing chunks of knowledge, clues into the male psyche that perhaps I'd previously overlooked or had never been exposed to. And I liked being able to share and explore new thinking with a *man*—a highly intelligent, experienced, older man—who also lived safely far away from me.

The bottom line was that, like it or not, a new door of my life was kicked open last summer. And it had led me to the chamber of my sexuality. I felt certain there were other doorways leading out of here, to other places; this wasn't my final destination. But before I could proceed onward, there was something hidden in here I had to find.

I AWOKE WITH a start, my bedroom dark and silent. *Geez, what time is it?* I looked over at my clock: 4:03 AM. The "birthing hours," an older spiritual teacher of mine had called these final hours before dawn. She'd said it was the perfect time to meditate; ripe earth energies were organizing themselves for the day ahead, and if one aligned herself, she could consciously create her day.

I rubbed my arms and stared at the ceiling. A dream had woken me and I remembered it vividly.

I was crouched down in front of my garden bed, digging up dead annuals with my trowel. Suddenly, I felt a tickle inside the arm of my long-sleeved shirt. I itched it and continued working. Awhile later, it happened again. I scratched and continued digging. *Ah, but my garden would be beautiful this year,* my dream self thought.

Then the tickles snuck up both arms at once. Maybe I had a rash? I sat back on my heels to take a peek. I rolled up my sleeves. *Oh, Christ!* My arms were covered with insects! I jumped up and vigorously started swiping them off. *Gross! Gross! Gross!*

Suddenly, a voice told me to calm down: *Look, Delaine, look at them.* Still panicked, I gazed down at my now totally bare arms. *Ladybugs. I'm covered in ladybugs.* Hundreds of them. I smiled. No need to be afraid. They were a reminder.

As I laid in bed remembering my dream, I rocked between

excitement and disbelief. *Ladybugs again. The ladybugs were back!* This had to be a sign, especially since I rarely remembered my dreams.

Back in March, one month before the Graham bomb went off, they had appeared in my dreams for the first time in my life. The dream was so unusual and emotional that I'd even told my girlfriends about it.

I was lying on a gynecologist table, legs spread, in preparation for my check-up. My doctor, a sixtyish woman with pulled-back gray hair and glasses, was busy on the other side of the room. All of a sudden, I felt something between my legs: movement, wiggling. *Worms!* I thought to myself, *I have worms—parasites!*

I screamed to the woman, "Help! Save me! them!" She looked over at me, totally unconcerned at all; instead, she seemed pleased.

I sat up and frantically looked down at my pelvis. *Hold on. Oh phew, they're not worms, they're ladybugs. This must be a dream.* I looked around the table and sheets. *Where the heck are they coming from?* I then watched, bewildered, as a stream of ladybugs emerged from my vagina. *What the!? Why were they in my VAGINA?* Then I woke up.

The dream was so bizarre yet vivid that the next morning I googled the meaning of a ladybug dream. I'd always felt akin to the Native American beliefs in animal totems; that is, each animal is symbolic and acts as a specific dream messenger. *What might a cute, red bug have to tell me?* I grinned.

Chills ran up and down my spine as I read about their meaning: *a sign of good luck, new beginnings, and rebirth.* My ladybugs had actually come out of my vagina. No doubt they were a sign of rebirth! This was too odd and loaded with meaning to be a coincidence, I thought. I took it as confirmation that I was on the right path, that a wonderful new chapter of my life was opening to me with Graham— that we were soul mates, destined to be together. It never occurred to me that rebirth required the death of something first.

Their reappearance tonight felt significant. I had experienced so much death! The death of love, the death of trust, and the death of my old self. At the cusp of so much change and uncertainty and second-guessing of myself, their return both soothed and uplifted me.

I curled my body into the fetal position with my hands cupped close to my chest. As I drifted off to sleep, I guarded the ladybugs' hope-filled message close to my heart.

CHAPTER 9

SERGEANT SHANE'S BOOT CAMP

THE DUKE SAID IT WAS time for me to "stop talking" and "start walking." It was time to get out of his online classroom and take action in the real world. He wrote:

> By the time you're finished overanalyzing everything, not only will the cows have come home, they'll have had babies, and their babies will have had babies. If you want to find and exert your alpha femaleness, you need to get out there.
>
> Think of it as having enlisted in a Sexuality Boot Camp, wherein I am your sergeant in command. Like a good little girl you will listen to your superior, and in turn, I'll make sure you keep your men in line—not to mention deliver good strong spankings when you're slacking off.
>
> What's that? Was that a "Yes Sir!"?

I laughed and thought, *How about "Bite me, sir."*

I leaned back in my chair, still smiling. *He sure does have a strange sense of humor.* But for whatever reason, *I liked it.* I liked that he caught me off guard, and I liked that he made me lighten up around the issue of dating and sex.

Shane's proposition appealed to me, despite the fact it was totally unconventional. Not taking every date seriously seemed a pretty sensible thing for me to do right now, because it liberated me to have fun and explore. Maybe my need to "seek and replace" wasn't as urgent as I once thought. Surely it wouldn't hurt to delay it a month or two . . .

I hit the reply button, smirking and shaking my head. *Yes, I think I'll play along with "Sergeant Shane."* Temporarily, anyway. Or unless Mr. Right comes along.

Mission No. 1
Subject's Name: Payton
Age: 36
Body Type: tall, average build
Penis Size: I've no clue, Shane!

My "training" kicked off with a wavy-haired computer techie named Payton. I reread Sergeant Shane's last directives before walking out the door to meet him:

> You can remain the classy good girl of old, but I want you to start thinking in terms of Dominant and submissive. No more settling for "nice." I don't want to hear about any more lukewarm nights. Let him know that any kissing will be decided by you. If you choose to see him again, he needs to know he will need to submit to your lead. If we're going to get you exploring this masculine side of you, you need to experiment a bit. You have no points on that side of the scoreboard yet.

I met Payton at a pub in his neighborhood, a twenty-minute drive from my house. As our date progressed, I willed myself to be interested in him. I couldn't quite finger why, but I wasn't attracted to him. *Give the guy a chance!* I barked at myself. *He's cute, he's smart, he's nice—what more do you want?*

But no matter how vigorously I rubbed my thoughts together, my body didn't spark.

Nonetheless, as per Shane's directives, I decided to "experiment" a bit near the end of our date, for curiosity's sake. Suddenly, the night didn't seem like just another disappointing, dead-end date.

Payton and I were in the parking lot, preparing for our final goodbyes. I could tell that he really wanted to kiss me, but earlier in the night, I had mischievously joked to him: "Don't even *think* about kissing me tonight without my permission. Otherwise I might just have to slap you."

Behind his half-smile, I could see him wondering, *Is she serious?*

I stood across from him in the parking lot, hands at my side, body language open. His eyes were darting, his hands fidgety: in his pockets, out of his pockets, through his hair, rubbing his chin. I could hear his thoughts, *Is she going to kiss me? God, I want to kiss her. Should I try to kiss her? Will she slap me?*

I stood where I was, staring at him unwaveringly. *Fidget-fidget squirm-squirm, fidget-fidget, squirm-squirm.* Outwardly I appeared cool and collected, but inwardly, my body surged with adrenaline. *Stay in control, Delaine,* I coached myself. *Stand in the tension. Don't back down.*

Finally, I smiled and offered him a handshake. "It was good to meet you, Payton. Thank you for the drink." And I turned and got in my minivan.

By the time I got home, my adrenaline rush was gone and I was convinced I'd just acted like a cold-hearted bitch. *You toyed with him like a cat does with a mouse,* I inwardly scolded. *Then why are you smiling?* taunted a voice in my head. *Admit it: it* was *kind of fun.*

I sat down at my computer, my smile quickly fading. Time to fill out a report. "Shane," I wrote. "No doubt I was in a dominant position tonight. But I have mixed feelings about my behavior. I can't help but wonder, Why am I doing this? What feeling am I striving for? In the big scheme of things, "playing" like this isn't sustainable."

To which he immediately replied:

Neither is laughing or eating chocolate cake or having a phenomenal orgasm. These things aren't 24/7, but they are a great way to make our lives a cabaret. So what if you don't want to see him again. Reject him, move on.

Let me remind you we're doing this because you want to explore your masculine side. This means you need to become comfortable feeling power. You had a small taste of it tonight. Don't run away from it because you're unfamiliar with it.

Just RELAX. God, sometimes you sound like the world is going to end tomorrow. You have thirty-seven years of how you have been, and we are seeking to explore another part of you. Don't expect the answer overnight. This isn't a fortune cookie.

His condescension was transparent and my blood quickly boiled. *How dare this jerk-off speak to me like I'm some kind of drama queen!*

But you are being a tad melodramatic, a part of me calmly stated. *He's just calling you out.* It suddenly dawned on me that maybe a good glove-slapping was what I needed. He was a Dom, not a sympathetic girlfriend—what, was I expecting him to rub my back and wipe away my tears? He and I were playing a *game*: sportsmanship rules required I toughen up.

My jets cooled off, I reread his message more objectively. *I* did *become aware of a new aspect of myself tonight,* I thought. It was kind of fun, too. Maybe I did need to stop worrying so much about what everyone else was thinking and feeling.

But this kind of power is calculated and potentially hurtful, a voice inside my head protested. *True power comes from treating everyone with love and respect.*

Oh, it's not like I beat the guy up or belittled him, I retorted. Don't be such a marshmallow, Delaine, he's *a big boy, not a child.*

I called a truce between my sensibilities and decided that, at least for now, I was going to study and play under Shane's tutelage—but *carefully.* Not only were other people's feelings at stake, so were mine.

A FEW DAYS later, I negotiated, signed, and sealed a deal with myself: I was placing my Internet business on the backburner. *Indefinitely.*

I'd stressed about it for months. Beat myself up for neglecting it. I'd poured my soul into that business; was *so* close to launching it. How could I just . . . walk away? Everyone would surely label me a quitter.

The bottom line was that pregnancy and childbirth and babies were of no interest to me. Given my recent life circumstances, the subject matter seemed like a twisted joke. And no matter how hard I willed myself to revive my passion for it, I felt nothing. Flat line.

A voice in my head objected, and rancorously: *You never finish anything! You bounce all over the place, there's a new flavor every day.* Those criticisms were too familiar; they first came from Robert. And now, even though he was gone, the tapes played automatically.

True, when I was younger, I never focused on just one job for very long. From renting out boogey boards and singing and playing guitar in the streets, to working in corporate finance and building a counseling business for women, my work life had taken some sudden swerves and detours.

But I never thought that was a *bad* thing. I just figured I had an adventurous spirit; that regardless of income earned (or not earned), each job was a life experience contributing to my being a more well-rounded and interesting person. I kind of liked that about me. I'd thought Robert did too.

But somewhere over the course of our marriage, he apparently "reassessed" my past and decided that it reflected "a very irresponsible, uncommitted person." More so, it made me "a spoiled little girl," always taking the liberty to do as I pleased.

I spent years wondering if he was right, doubting myself and my character. Maybe without a man's steady financial support, I'd be in for a huge reality jolt. Maybe I really was a spoiled brat. I knew I couldn't earn the same amount as him in the workforce, especially the longer I stayed out of it. I felt indebted to Robert: All those long hours and weeks he spent away from home were for me and the kids, he'd remind me; "I'd work a fraction of the time if it were just me," he'd say. I was wracked with guilt; after all, I enjoyed my life as a stay-at-home mom. His suffering was for my gain.

Almost all my mom friends had returned to work within a year of giving birth. To a "real job," Robert called it. "Not everyone has the luxury of staying home all day, eating bon-bons, and watching Oprah." He was so off—and I tried to explain the scope and value of my hard work at home. But he cut me off: "Geez, you women never stop complaining. My grandma had six kids, no appliances, and she had to grow our food and work in the fields. Maybe I should've married a good ol' farm girl." No matter how I tried to explain my situation to him, it fell on deaf ears. "Every uterus has been doing what you do since the beginning of time," he joked backhandedly. "C'mon Delaine. Cowboy up."

So I did. I saddled up and shut up. I knew how tough a job I had, I knew how hard I worked. *He just doesn't understand the demands of parenting because he works out of town*, I told myself. *But that's okay. I'm strong and I don't need his validation.*

I knew he was wrong in his assessment of my past, too. I had finished six years of university, held two lengthy professional jobs, *but . . . but . . .*

The seeds of self-doubt had taken root. The Delaine I saw reflected back through his eyes was much less than what I'd credited her to be. I knocked myself down a few notches. Then a few more.

In hindsight, I can actually *see* the slow destruction of my sense of self over the years. His words, like sharp pins, covered my body from head to toe like a well-used voodoo doll. I'd thought my skin was tough and thick. But his attacks were too numerous. Slowly, his toxic criticisms had poisoned my sense of self-worth.

I could *not* allow Robert to call the shots on my life anymore! I *knew* this, but it was a lot easier said than done. His verbal pins had transformed into arrows since we'd separated. We were still disagreeing over a few important points on our separation agreement, particularly those related to money. Any time Robert and I entered discussion around it, I could literally see the anger climb up his back and ignite a fire in his eyes, burning out his ability to reason. Suddenly, we were no longer talking about the issue at hand, and all my energy went into shielding off his attacks on my character:

"You were nothing but a footloose hippie before you met me. And you'd *still* be nothing if it weren't for me!"

"I see you're on the dating sites, God, what a joke. You describe yourself as athletic . . . smart? You're the most fucked-up woman I've ever known!"

"You think I'm not paying you enough? Well, how about if I work only half-time and take the kids the other half? Then you won't get *anything!*"

I knew Robert was hurting. I also knew he was afraid. And I *did* feel compassion for him: He was processing the death of our marriage, too. But I didn't know where to draw the line around his taking out his pain on me; there was no pleasure in being the victim of his verbal assaults, but there was also no pleasure in seeing him suffering and upset. Moreover, what if I was WRONG? What if I was acting selfishly, but didn't see it?

So I'd just wrap my arms tightly around my chest, imagine myself wrapped in white light, and take it.

But *no more*. I knew it was time to *stop* taking it, to *stop* justifying my life to Robert, and focus on being true to me. Suddenly, Shane's voice replayed in my ears: "From now on, you let no one disrespect you, even *you* . . . You're no one's doormat anymore. You got that?"

The "alpha" in me stirred. I got it alright. I had gotten rid of Robert, the flesh and blood man; *now* I needed to cauterize the wounds he'd left in my soul.

CHAPTER 10
MANEUVERS AND TOUCHDOWNS

I WAS KEEPING A SECRET from Sergeant Shane. Nothing shocking or scandalous. But I knew he would think I was being naughty for not telling him.

Turns out, I met someone online I actually liked. Maybe even more than Shane. And I'd been sneaking out of boot camp to see him.

His name was Chad. He was the fresh-faced quarterback look-alike who emailed me the night of my sex-club adventure. For whatever reason, he didn't write me again until a few days ago. But we'd quickly made up for lost time.

As it turned out, my intuition was spot-on: He looked like a jock because he *was* a jock. Not only was he a high school physical education teacher, he was also the school's football coach. He had no kids of his own, but his students served as surrogates; he spent countless volunteer hours with his athletes after school and spoke passionately about the issues teenagers faced, including the confusion, adventures, and heartbreak of adolescence.

Part of his teaching curriculum also required he teach sex education to his gym students. And though we sometimes shared a giggle at their telltale awkwardness or bravado, my jaw fell open when he shared the inside scoop on some students' escapades:

Some teenagers, he said, proudly wear bracelets that mark the number of sexual partners they'd had at weekend parties. Some also engaged in "rainbow parties," where girls compete in a contest of sorts—performing oral sex on boys while wearing different color lipstick, thus creating a rainbow. "They announce their sexual exploits as if it somehow makes them cool," said Chad. "If I were a parent, I'd be looking at my child's wrist *very* carefully."

I suddenly felt like I'd been living in a bubble for the past twenty years. Back in the eighties, I thought my friends and I were being promiscuous when we smoked a joint and got felt-up in someone's bathroom. But engaging in sex for sport? Suddenly, I wanted to shackle my kids!

For our first date, Chad invited me to go shopping to buy his mom a birthday present. Out front of the wholesale store, we finally met face to face; there was direct eye contact and big smiles on both sides. I liked what I saw. His face was handsome yet boyish, his small brown eyes and long eyelashes shimmered with mischief, and his white-toothed smile stretched from ear to ear. Like me, he was wearing jeans and a casual shirt. But his was a red and white football jersey—and *whew*, there was no denying the broad, muscular chest it concealed.

We meandered side by side toward the jewelry department, talking and laughing like old pals. Along the way, we checked out flat-screen TVs and a few deluxe barbeques (I feigned interest). The whole date-while-shopping experience felt pleasant, but very odd, especially since I'd wheeled through this store a hundred times with my kids.

He'd already narrowed his gift search down to two items: a diamond teardrop pendant and a diamond-laced gold bracelet. "Which would you prefer?" he asked, pointing them out in the showcase.

As I bent forward to examine his selections, Chad leaned over the top of me, with his hand on my waist. I made no effort to move away from the warm press of his body, which immediately aroused me. For an intense moment I forgot I was shopping . . . *Yoo-hoo, Delaine, make a choice!* "Definitely the bracelet." And our bodies separated.

A couple of hotdogs and sodas later, we wrapped up our date with a big strong hug (against his big strong chest) and his declaration to call me soon. Overall, our date left me feeling pumped and ready to square off with him again. The idea of being tackled was *very* appealing.

LOST IN THE warm thoughts of my date with Football Coach Chad, I began walking home from the grocery store. Even though my five grocery bags were heavy, I decided to take the longer, scenic route through the park. It was a beautiful day, and besides, I needed the exercise.

Halfway into the park, I stopped and put down my bags to rest my numbing arms. It was then that I noticed someone lying down on the far side of the hill.

I froze, my heart kicking into high gear. He had a long body and short, dark hair. I clenched the handles of my grocery bags and walked slowly in his direction, feeling pulled, *pushed,* as if under a spell. Eyes straight ahead, I proceeded through the large evergreens. Fifteen feet away now, out of the trees and into the buttery afternoon sunlight . . .

It was HIM. He was lying where we used to picnic during his lunch hours. Still, I continued moving toward him, silently, not even a faint rustle from my bags. I felt like I was floating ghostlike, as if I was astral-traveling to "here," to this moment, to this Netherland of my past. I stopped right beside him and looked down. He was sleeping.

"Hi Graham," I said, in a voice colder than I intended.

He quickly sat up and removed his sunglasses. "Oh geez—you scared me!"

Pause.

"How *are* you?" he asked hesitantly.

"Good . . . . and you?"

"I'm okay." He moved over on his blanket to make room for me to sit down. I ignored the gesture and stood there gripping my grocery bags. I wanted to look down on him. I felt strangely unmoved.

"How's your business going?" he asked.

"It's not. I've had too much else to deal with." He looked away.

"How's work for you?" I asked.

"Not good. I'm not sure what's going on. I've gone from having a three-week waiting list to having hours off every day. All I know is that it's the beginning of the month and I have eighty dollars in my bank account."

"Wow." I stared down at him, feeling no pity. *Sucks when karma catches up with you, eh?*

I knew he was now the father of a four-month-old baby girl; my friend Sara had informed me the day she'd been born. Right now, I wasn't about to pretend that she and her mother never happened.

"Do you get to see your daughter very much?" I asked directly.

He paused, fiddling with his glasses. When he finally spoke, he did not look at me. "Usually once a week."

I nodded slowly. I could tell from his demeanor that the truth had not yet surfaced, that he was still doing damage control. Because you see, Melissa, his girlfriend/friend/lover or whatever she was, was *married*; not only that, she had four other kids from this marriage. And her husband, even though he'd had a vasectomy two years ago, believed the baby she'd just birthed was *his*. That's right. Graham and Melissa had knowingly stood by and allowed her husband to fall in love with another man's child. They resorted to sneak visits behind her husband's back, and they had yet to formulate a long-term game plan . . . somebody, at some point, was going to be devastated.

As I looked down at Graham now, sitting in a long-sleeved polo shirt on this hillside full of intimate memories, I felt strangely calm and composed. He looked the same as he always had—but somehow . . . . somehow . . . he felt like a stranger; I knew him, yet I did not. I had pressed against that lean chest in the throes of our lovemaking. I had excavated and shared my innermost thoughts and dreams with him. I had planned to love his three children and build my entire future with HIM—this man, this stranger, sitting on a blanket, in the afternoon sunshine.

"So Graham—" I looked him straight in the eyes. "Do you have any regrets?" I felt the power behind my question hit Graham square in the chest like a well-placed punch.

He flinched, I swear, and his chiseled jaw dropped. He did not expect that question, either. At first he looked pained, and then his eyes flashed with defensiveness. "I have no regrets for bringing my daughter into this world. She is beautiful and I would never regret giving her life." Then his tone softened. "But . . . I do regret all the people I hurt."

I nodded my head, mouth tight. *Was that supposed to be an apology? You still have no balls, you selfish coward.*

"Well, I need to get going." I rustled my grocery bags. "Good-bye, Graham."

"Bye, Delaine. It was great to see you."

I started walking away. "Hey Delaine," he called. I turned around. "Thanks for stopping. Thanks for talking to me."

"Bye, Graham." I turned my back to him, and with my head held high, I walked across the remaining length of the open park. I knew I was visible to him the entire way. I knew he was watching me leave, hoping I'd look back over my shoulder. But I didn't. I didn't even want to. And that said it all.

It was Saturday night, a week since my first date with Coach Chad. Even though Chad was at a wedding reception, he'd texted me numerous times throughout the evening. And it was clear that he was becoming increasingly inebriated. But that was okay, because so was I.

After a month on the road, Robert had unexpectedly come to town and taken the kids for twenty-four hours. And I was beyond ecstatic. Oh, I love my kids more than anything, but as any busy mother will attest, me-time is a rare treasure. When I look back on the last seven years of my life, I'm baffled by where my energy came from; hell, how did my engine even turn over some days? Even when Robert was in town to help out, my workload didn't lessen, it simply changed. His short returns home meant a mad rush to maximize the ever-important family time that most other families share on a regular basis. Plus, I had to organize fun husband-wife date nights—not just dinners out (which I preferred), but dancing, bars, live bands, *action*. "Just because you're a mom doesn't mean you have to act like an old lady," he'd say, if I protested. I didn't want to be perceived as *that* kind of wife: Mrs. I-Am-Boring-and-No-Fun, now that I've had kids. No—it was my duty to maintain my pre-mom vibrancy and be the same energetic woman Robert fell in love with, even though I longed to be treated like a lady and not his party girl . . . or maybe just fall asleep on the couch.

Robert took the kids too late in the day for me to make plans to go out. So instead, I caught up with a few girlfriends via phone and, as usual, chatted online. I'd been corresponding with a few young men, who were between twenty-seven and thirty, for a couple of weeks now. Just harmless flirting, with no real agenda . . . yet.

Around eight o'clock, I cracked open a bottle of white wine—which I'd never done alone (kids have no sympathy for a hung-over parent)—and poured myself a generous glass. Tonight I didn't have to worry about getting up with the kids, and I was filled with restless energy. After my texting repartee with Chad, I was hoping, even expecting him to call or drop by after the reception. But in the meantime, I'd happily throw a private party—for just Me, Myself and I.

As I sat at my desk, my wine buzz quickly kicking in, I discovered a trove of online music videos that I'd never had time to watch. Shakira, Rihanna, the Dixie Chicks, Madonna—*damn!*—when did they start writing songs based on *my* life? Belting out their lyrics was no longer enough: I moved my office chairs off to the side and *voila!*—instant dance floor. What started as a few hip rolls with a well-balanced wine glass in hand turned into full-blown, full-body, Mom-Going-Nuts in her SuperGirl pajama bottoms and bra (I got sweaty!). Anyone watching me would have thought "Wow, what an ass," but as I caught my reflection in the picture frames on the wall, all I could think was *YEAH, you still got the moves girl! Pfft, if Robert and Graham could see me now!* And as I inwardly cursed my former husband and lover I suddenly wished they could see who I was becoming, who they were missing out on: a woman on the verge—not of a nervous breakdown, but of a break*through*. Metamorphosis. Because I *liked* this new, emerging Delaine, now that she was out of their shadows. I *liked* the fact that I was drunk by myself and dancing around half-naked at home on a Saturday night. I *liked* the fact that younger men wanted to jump in bed with me. I *liked* feeling sexy and desirable . . . and a little wild, and a lot horny. God, I was *so* grateful I wasn't sitting across from Graham in a makeshift house with our six children squeezed into shared beds. Or kowtowing to Robert, as he belittled me and further killed my self-worth, not to mention my sexuality. Well, fuck them and the horses (or women) they rode in on! Life was just getting good for me . . . With my head beginning to feel spinny, I hit the hay—keeping my phone next to me, just in case Football Coach Chad called . . .

Sure enough, the sound of a text mail interrupted my hazy sleep. I squinted at the bright cell phone screen, trying to focus on the little black letters that jumped out at me: "U awake? Comin ovr? 1632 Blackbird Dr."

I glanced at my clock: 1:45 AM. I quickly texted back: "Give me 30 mins."

A couple minutes later, my phone bleeped again: "Come on in. Door open."

So this was probably not the smartest decision. A rendezvous at a man's house in the middle of the night meant only one thing. And a first time I'm-drunk-and-horny encounter could very well set the stage for it being a last encounter. Men need to work for it, don't they? Wine you, dine you, respect you? But I wasn't interested in deciphering anyone else's "rules"—I liked him, I was sick of due diligence, and I wanted to have sex.

Forty minutes later, after freshening up, brushing my teeth ten times, and Mapquesting directions to his house, I pulled up in front of his bungalow. All the neighbors' houses were dark and quiet, as was Chad's, except for a dim light coming from a back room. I stepped into the chilly night wearing my winter jacket and my Super Girl jammies underneath. I'd packed some clothes for the morning.

I walked right in, as per his instructions. In the dark foyer, a wet nose pressed against my hand. It was his golden retriever, Buddy. *Hey there.* Pat, pat. *Where's your master?* His tail banged against the wall.

I took off my jacket and laid it on the couch. I stood there, expecting Chad to walk into the room or at least call out to me. But only Buddy seemed to know I was there.

"Chad?" I called out softly. No answer.

"Chad?" I called again, walking through to the kitchen where a dim light glowed. Still no answer. With my hands tracing the wall, I began shuffling down a long dark corridor.

Finally, I came to a room at the end of the hall with its door ajar. My eyes were adjusting to the dark, and I could make out the shape of a bed in the corner. I listened for a second and heard heavy, slow breathing. He was passed out! I stood there trying to decide what to do. Was this a sign to leave?

Oh screw it! I thought, as I walked over to the bed, pulled back the covers, and slid in beside him. He was naked.

"What the—" he chuckled gruffly. He pulled me tightly into a spoon and I snuggled in close. "Am I dreaming or did a beautiful woman just jump into bed with me in the middle of the night?" His hands firmly traced down the side of my body.

"No, you're not dreaming," I laughed. "Problem is, you're passed out."

"Yeah, guess I dozed off a bit." He lifted the covers off me. "What are you wearing?"

"My Super Girl pajamas."

"Ah, yes. The infamous Super Girl PJs. Sooooo sexy. But—" He pulled me underneath him—strong arms, thick muscular body. "I think they need to come *off*." He kissed me. And for the next hour, this girl felt pretty darn super.

IN THE REALM of lovemaking, there are "bad lovers" and "good lovers," and then there are "knock-your-socks-off, knee-wobbling lovers." As good luck would have it—and I'm talking major windfall here—Chad fell into the latter category. Not only was he sensual and generous, his skill set was beyond excellent—so much so that my body did something it's never done before . . .

Now, up to this point, I thought I knew my body very well. I'd lived in it for thirty-seven years, bore three little humans from it, pushed it to its physical limits. And while I'd never, say, participated in a rainbow blowjob competition, I'd certainly had my fair share of sexual experiences, so I thought I knew what would make me orgasm, how I liked to be touched, and *how my body would respond to such touch* . . . I considered myself a pretty knowledgeable and experienced lover. But *whoa*, was I wrong! Chad had me doing things I'd never done before *and* my body shocked me by reacting in a brand new way. Not only did I G-spot orgasm for the first time, I did something else: I squirted (queue me cringing a little after admitting this).

Now clearly, the term itself is enough to make anyone squirm. Something about the idea of shooting warm liquid out of your lady parts during orgasm can seem, well, *un*ladylike. In fact, it may be a subject that's too personal, even off-putting, for some women to handle—like discussing the nuances of getting a Brazilian wax (how *do* you keep your inner labia from getting scorched by hot wax, anyway?). Squeamishness aside, I was absolutely stunned when my body did this. And not once, but several times.

Squirting was something I knew very little about it. I mean, I'd *heard* of it. But I'd thought it sounded *freaky*.

This was one for my girlfriends; I definitely needed their input. Imagine my surprise when I discovered that about a quarter of them had experienced what I thought was a rare phenomenon. *Women aren't supposed to ejaculate,* I thought. But apparently, we are. And further, each woman experienced it differently: some with deep penetration, some with oral stimulation. But it wasn't consistent, they said; there wasn't a *formula* for it. Sometimes it happened, more often it didn't. But they all agreed on one thing: When it did happen, it felt great.

During my first orgasm (there were many), Chad was sitting upright on his knees and I was on my back with my hips up high. Nothing unusual about this position. But then he started with the "Chad Maneuver," a technique that broke the dam.

He took hold of his penis (average size) and slipped it in about two inches. Then, with just the right pressure, he started vigorously rubbing himself up and down inside me. At first, I thought, *What the heck is he DOING?* But after a few seconds, it started to feel incredible. I couldn't help but moan and surrender to the sensation. Suddenly, I started to orgasm, and while in the throes I heard, "Oh yeah baby, you're squirting!" I felt a huge release and wetness sprayed all over him *and* me. A part of me wanted to *say* something at that point, but I was too shocked and weak to do more than just lie there smiling.

Our session was far from over. Chad then thrust deep inside me for a minute or so and then started with his maneuver again (two inches in, vigorous rubbing). The feeling came back so quick and intense, that I sprayed again . . . and again . . . and *again.*

Afterward, the bed was too wet to lay on—the sheets *and* the mattress. I apologized profusely for my mess as we covered the mattress with towels and remade the bed. He teased, "Why didn't you tell me you were a squirter?"

"Because I've never been one before!" I said, laughing.

"Really?"

"Yes, I swear that has never happened to me before!"

"Well, cool. Now you know you can." He was smiling and seemed comfortable with what had transpired. I, on the other hand, was embarrassed, as if I had just bled all over his sheets from my period. As we climbed back into our newly made bed and snuggled up close, I had questions:

"Have you been with other women who squirted?"

"Yes. Maybe five." *Thank God. So he doesn't think I'm abnormal.*

"So . . . it's pretty common then?"

"Well no, not really."

"Hmmm . . . " *Guess I'm still part of the borderline "freaky" group.*

"So you mean that in all those years you were married, you never squirted?" he asked.

"No, *never!* In fact, I remember my ex-husband telling me once that he'd seen it on a porno and he wished that I *could.*" Chad chuckled. I continued: "That 'maneuver' you did on me was sensational. No one's ever done that to me before."

"Well it obviously worked on you." He was being modest, but I could tell he was pleased.

"I think you should give classes on it and teach the rest of the male population how to do it," I blurted.

"It doesn't seem like all that big a secret. It just makes sense to me. Once a woman's all warmed up, the G-spot is located just a couple of inches inside. I can position myself at the right angle to stimulate it. It often helps if I also put pressure on the outside of her pubic bone with my hand."

"You were touching the front of my pubic bone?" (*Too busy feeling sensations elsewhere.*)

"Yeah," he laughed. "Almost the entire time."

"Hmmm. So did that 'maneuver' feel good for you, too?"

"Yeah, it was GREAT. I had to stop myself from orgasming the first time you squirted."

I sighed blissfully and snuggled in closer.

Then he added: "We'll have to try it again in the morning and find out if it was just a fluke."

And we did. With sunlight streaming in through the windows, he made me orgasm and squirt half a dozen more times. One time, he even did it with his *fingers.*

"Holy Toledo, Chad!" I said as we changed the sheets again. "Now you're *really* impressing me. What the heck were you doing in there?"

He just laughed.

"Um . . . I'm serious." I stopped mid sheet-change and put my hands on my hips. "I want to know how you did that with your fingers."

"It's pretty straight forward, really. You know how the G-spot is supposed to be activated with the 'come here' motion—" He bent his index and middle fingers to demonstrate. I nodded. "I find it works better when you do 'come here' combined randomly with a 'go up.' And it has to be done pretty hard, not gently." He demonstrated the combination of movements in front of his face—fingers were a flyin': *Up- up-up, curl-curl, up, curl-curl, up . . .* "Just tell guys to imagine they're playing a trumpet." We laughed.

Over the next hour, we showered, had breakfast, and leisurely talked and hung out. I didn't want to overstay my welcome, so I volunteered to leave on my own. He hugged and kissed me goodbye, and as I floated to my car in the brisk autumn air, he waved to me in the doorway.

As I made my way home, basking in the glow of amazing uninhibited sex, I couldn't help but wonder, *Why the heck did my squirting happen now?* Why not with Graham? After all, we'd *made love*. But instead of letting loose with the man I believed to be the love of my life, it happened with a guy I hardly knew! That made no sense to me. Was it a function of my pent-up sexual frustration? Or my age and that I was done having children? Or was I becoming more in tune with my body? But that didn't make any sense either—I'd been treating my body horribly, not eating, smoking cigarettes, not sleeping. *God, I felt like such a newbie!*

Suddenly, a new thought zoomed in for landing: *Maybe the "why" doesn't matter.* What if I wasn't supposed to understand why it happened. Maybe my body was simply ready. Maybe I was simply meant to *enjoy the experience.* No "because," just *period.*

Gosh, was such a thing even possible?

All I knew for sure was that I was thrilled by this unexpected "gift"—kind of like looking down and discovering a treasure box sitting on my lap—or in my case, between my legs. I was flooded with sudden gratitude: If I'd stayed married to Robert, I'd never have experienced anything like this; my sexual self would've remained in lockdown. When Graham came along, reigniting my sexual energy and bringing me to new heights of lovemaking, I'd thought my sexual evolution had reached the final pinnacle; that every other experience would be downhill from there; that I'd be struggling to recreate what I once had . . . and lost. Instead, not only did I feel more personally liberated, I'd discovered a whole new aspect of my sexuality that I never knew existed. And it was empowering! Because it was *my* body that experienced it. And it suggested that there was more to me, more to sex, more to my *life* than I'd ever realized. I felt *hopeful* . . . Maybe all the emptiness that sorrow had gutted into my bones this past year would one day spill over with happiness.

Because why shouldn't a profound sexual experience be any less contemplated as a life catalyst than "making love"? Isn't making love but an ideal that we use to validate sex, as if the pleasure our bodies experience is not, in itself, worthy on its own? We cloak the act of sex in the chastity of love to play down the carnal, as if carnal is wrong. But why? Certainly, religion, social conditioning, gender stereotyping, culture, etc., play a role here (control, anyone?), but I wanted to blast aside those filters and honor the rawness of the experience for what it was: a *pure* expression of my Sexual Self, which was an intimate aspect of who I was as a woman—yet someone I'd consistently mistrusted in the past. What if this was actually an honest and wise aspect of myself that I'd been ignoring? Maybe "she" could direct me down new avenues of joy and pleasure. Maybe she was a powerful conduit of creativity—even epiphanies—that could be applied to other areas of my life.

The only thing I knew for sure was that I wanted to investigate her further . . .

CHAPTER 11

OPERATION SERVICE BOY(S)

"SO HAVE YOU HEARD FROM Chad?" Hali asked me over the phone. It was Thursday, four days since Chad and I had spent our first (soaking wet) night together.

"No, but I'm not surprised. He said his weeknights are crazy-busy right now with the football team. It's all good."

"Fair enough. You're good for a little while anyway, eh?" she teased.

"Yes!" I enthused. I was *still* smiling. "What about you? Any fireworks on your date last night with the lawyer?"

"Nah. He was nice and everything, but he looked so *old*. That photo he posted on the site is way too flattering. He's only forty-three but he's an *old* forty-three."

"Oh, Hali!" I laughed at her bluntness, but I also felt guilty; I had been harshly judging men online by their physical appearance, too. And I worried this made me shallow. After all, everyone has flaws, everyone gets older, and it wasn't like I was a supermodel.

"I know it sounds awful to say," Hali continued, "but there really is a big difference in how people age. I don't think commenting on it is being superficial; it's just the obvious truth. You and I were both married to young, attractive, athletic men; that's the ideal we're used to, and that's what we like." Then softly: "And wow, Paul really looks amazing these days . . ."

Warning bells went off in my head. Paul and his "soul mate" had broken up a few weeks ago, and though he wasn't actively trying to win Hali back, I knew she was still vulnerable to him. Before I had a chance to express my concern, Hali changed the subject: "I'm just so damn horny and aware of my sexuality these days. The other day I was grocery shopping with the kids, and you know what I started doing? *The stripper walk.* The one I learned in my stripping class."

I burst out laughing. "As you walked up the aisles?"

"Yes! Through the produce section, too. I even had Teah strapped to my chest in the Baby Bjorn while I did it."

I laughed even harder.

She continued: "And you know what? It really worked! Men were looking at me."

"I've no doubt they *were.*" I wiped away tears. "Ohhh, man. Thanks for the laugh. So tell me, what *is* the stripper walk anyway?"

"The most important thing to remember is that each time you take a step, place your foot directly in front of the other. This is key because it makes your rear-end wiggle more. And men *love* the sway of a woman's hips and butt."

"'K, you'll have to show me when I see you next. Speaking of, what are you doing this weekend? You're without kids, right?"

"Yeah. Josh is working, and I'm all alone. And it sucks because I really want to get laid. Got a man for me?" She made an attempt to laugh, but I could tell it was forced. This wasn't just about wanting sex; she was hurting.

Two weeks ago, Paul had started taking both kids every second weekend, instead of just her older son. Hali had phoned me in tears shortly after he picked them up: "It's just not fair! God, I didn't think it would be so hard to hand Teah over to him. She's just so young and small, she's *my* baby girl. While he was out fucking his girlfriend, I was carrying her and giving birth to her and loving and caring for her. And when she looked up at me from her car seat with those big, beautiful, innocent eyes, my heart was in my throat as I gave her to him. It took everything in me not to snatch her back, to not scream at him, *'Give me back my baby! You don't fucking deserve her!'* But I held it together for the kids' sake. I smiled and gave him all the baby supplies he'd need for the weekend. But as soon as I shut the front door, I sat on the floor in the entryway and bawled for twenty minutes."

I'd listened to her with an ache in my heart. *God, when does the pain end? When will "living" require less of us?* I reminded her that "first times" are always the hardest; that it would get easier—it *had* to.

But Hali had never enjoyed spending large chucks of time alone. Now she was alone for entire weekends. If she didn't fill them up with friends and activities, she'd stay in her pajamas and succumb to depression.

She needed some distraction, and at times like this, comfort in the form of a strong set of shoulders and a big penis really come in handy. "Hali," I said. "Do you remember that guy Don I dated one time, about a month ago? I thought he was a player—the bed-post-notcher that looked like a shorter Val Kilmer? Maybe I could set you two up this weekend. As long as you understand it will probably be a one-nighter."

"You met him in person, right? You thought he was cute?"

"Yes! And he's got a pretty hot 'bad boy' air about him." I filled her in on a few more details. Finally, "I think you guys could have a lot of fun together."

"Oh what the hell, why not."

A few minutes later, I dug up Don's last email and got to work. *What are friends for, right?*

Unfortunately, the weekend passed without either of us getting distracted by a penis, let alone a strong set of shoulders. But

Hali and bad-boy Don *did* start chatting, and the sexual innuendoes were flying. Systems engaged, engines running, the countdown to their sexual launch had begun.

As for me, Football Coach Chad hadn't called yet. *What the hell? Now* I was feeling a little jilted. We'd had great sex and got along fabulously. My mind raced with excuses for him: Maybe he was busy with family or school or his volunteer work. Or maybe he was playing it cool because he liked me *too* much.

Whatever the reasons, it hurt my pride. I was *not* going to sit around waiting for him, or any other man for that matter. I waited around too long for Graham. Never again! To hell with Chad. *Stupid jock.*

Grumbling, I fired up my computer to check my mail on the Sugar Daddy site. Ahhh, a message from Shane:

> Where's my next date report?
> We need to work with this phenomenon of the young
> boys liking you. You've been kind of surprised by the
> young-boy attention, so perhaps not mentally prepared
> for it. In general, boys like this should be submissive to
> you. But we need to figure out what your brain looks like
> so we can work with it.

I leaned back in my chair, Coach Chad forgotten. What *do* I think of younger-male attention? *Is* this something I want to explore?

Because being promiscuous with young men didn't blend with the image I had of who I was: caring, upstanding neighbor on the block; loving, dedicated mother to three children; smart business woman who was also a lady. I believed I was a woman who conducted her life by high principles and morals, and slutting around with young boy toys was NOT me. It was Madonna.

Someone once told me you should pretend a video camera is

following you every minute of the day. And if you wouldn't want what you're doing to be broadcast to the masses, it's probably wrong.

Pffft, that's ridiculous! a voice retorted in my head. *Everyone has sex and most don't want it broadcast to the world. That doesn't make casual sex wrong!* No—just because I was a divorced mom didn't mean I had to stay home every night, alphabetize my spice rack, and plot my kids' futures. I was a mature woman who had sexual wants and needs, just like any other normal, healthy person. *Geez, I finally get rid of my bullyish husband and yet I'm still following someone else's rule book*, I thought, irritated.

But what was the alternative? Write my own? I wasn't convinced I was strong enough to go against the herd. Nor was I certain I could trust myself.

I sighed and glanced over at Shane's email: young-man attention. *If I* did *choose to follow Shane's directives and play with, maybe even dominate, a young lover or two, the bottom line was that no one else needed to know. I wasn't sixteen anymore, I knew how to keep a secret.*

But what if I'm fooling myself into trivializing sex? What if the main reason why people are sexually attracted to one another is nature's way of ensuring we constantly seek to bond with, care for, and love someone?

Oh PUULLEEZE. Would you STOP?! I scolded. Who *was* this overly chaste person, anyway? Unfortunately, it was *me*—conditioned so well about how a woman/wife/mother should and should not behave, that my *ability* to be self-expressive had been genuinely stifled. Growing up, the messages I heard about sexuality were that only in marriage would I feel safe enough, comfortable enough, to fully explore the fire of my sexuality; it was supposed to automatically come with the territory of true love, right? But I wondered how many women truly found their marital sex life as prolific and satisfying as they'd imagined it would be? Like me, how many wished their husbands would intuitively know how to touch them, seduce them, and romance them, without having to spell it out to them? And how many of us even knew *how* to? Over time, did most women make it a priority to voice their hidden wants and desires? Or did their fire get dowsed by inhibitions that deemed such desires as unimportant, selfish, or worse, somehow *deviant?* For many, including me, submissiveness—by default, not choice, both in and out of bed—was a condition of marriage.

Perhaps this was why I couldn't recall having any burning sexual wants and curiosities during my marriage, even at the beginning, when we couldn't keep our hands off each other. I believed I was pretty uninhibited, and the sex was physically fulfilling. But the aftermath of sex and the joy of being in love meant as much, if not more to me: the cuddling, the pillow-talk, the dream of one day having children and building a life together. To me, sex was just a small part of the "us" equation. Independent of Robert, it was anything but a priority to me.

The truth was, I never really pondered what sex meant to *me.* I knew I had sexual impulses; "animal urges" in need of appeasement. But not once did I think of my Sexual Self as being an important aspect of my Spiritual Self. Not once did I think of it as a source of *my* beauty, *my* creative expression, *my* empowerment. Never did it cross my mind that my sexual passion—or lack thereof—might be partially shaping the overall composition of Delaine.

The bottom line was that I had fire in me *right now,* I thought, as I returned to Shane's email. And there was no inkling of a love relationship on the horizon. So I had to decide: Was I going to smolder the fire? Keep it safely under control? Or was I going to play with it, blend with it, maybe even dance naked around it, and see if it was something worth celebrating?

Decision made, I logged onto the dating site and pulled up the profiles of two young men who had hunted me for weeks: Daniel and Brent. I wrote them asking for their chat addresses. *Time to find out if there'd be any combustion.*

Next I responded to Shane's email, briefly outlining my intentions and action plan. At the end, on impulse, I added: "It's really quite fun corresponding with you, Shane. In not knowing your identity or seeing your face, I kinda feel like you're my 'Charlie' from Charlie's Angels."

I fired it off into cyberspace, imagining a man with thick hairy forearms and a gold watch reading it at his desk with a smile.

The next morning Shane's reply was waiting in my inbox:

There is a term I have for men like your prospects: "service males." They are hot, well-endowed males who are essentially walking dildos. They are not relationship material, but fun to f*** under the right circumstances.

These young boys will be too young for you to care about or spend non-sex time with. Talking to a service male is like talking to a puppy. They aren't for talking to. They are little boys, not men to rely on. Just put boys like this in their place, use them how YOU want, then kick their ass out the door until you want them again (if ever). If they cry about wanting to see you again, tell them to shut the f*** up and you'll let them know if you want to use them in the future. In the meantime, they can wash your car.

Re "Charlie": I'm glad you're loosening up. Stop sweating the trivia. I prefer to think of myself as a SAM—Super Alpha Male. Sam can prepare the alpha female to eventually bond with another alpha male or mentally hold her hand while she dominates the submissive. As much

Yes, Charlie! Er, I mean SAM or Duke or Shane, or whoever you are.

I sat back in my chair and reread his message. *Service males? Super Alpha Male?* Where did he even come up with such terms?

But in a weird way, I was grateful to have him on my team; he was a knowledgeable and caring guardian/protector of sorts. And it felt good knowing that no matter how far I pushed the boundaries, he'd be on my side, "watching over me" from afar.

I just hoped my guardian angels weren't panicking.

Mission No. 2
Subject's Name: Adonis-Boy Daniel
Age: 27
Body Type: 6 feet tall and ripped from head to toe
Penis Size: 6 ½ inches

Right from the get-go with Daniel, I decided that *I* was going to call the shots. Even during our preliminary email exchanges, I wrote things I'd never dare say face-to-face. One email he wrote: "I may only be twenty-seven, but I can make your toes curl and you scream my name."

To which I responded: "Hon, there isn't a man who walks the face of this planet who doesn't think he's 'all that' in bed. Until I say otherwise, you are not to even think about me in a sexual way. You haven't *earned* it. And if you want to play to my thought in the future, you need to ask for my permission." (I got that idea from Shane.)

His response: "I humbly place myself at your feet, Oh Master. Lol, you sound like a lot of fun!"

As I sat across from him at our initial meeting, I was impressed. He was smart, well-spoken and . . . oh, who am I trying to kid? The guy was absolutely gorgeous! His teeth were perfectly white, his hair thick and blond, his intense green eyes almost laugh-line free. I found myself trying to mentally sketch a composite of how he'd look at my age. *Yep, still strikingly handsome*—even with the goatee he was currently sporting (which I'm not normally a fan of).

So yes, the spark was definitely there for me at our first meeting. But I wasn't sure if it was mutual. *What if he thought I looked old? Did he tell the waitress I was his aunt when I went to the bathroom? Did he see me as the other dreaded C-word—COUGAR?*

Who could blame me for being insecure. He was Greek god Adonis in a snowboard T-shirt, and I was a single mother, ten years his senior.

I didn't *want* to care so darn much about what any man thought of me, whatever his age. But, like my role as chaste wife/mother, it was pretty ingrained, this need for validation of my desirability. That's why I liked this bizarre arrangement with Shane. It pushed me to be tougher about how I managed my dating/sex life. It challenged me *not* to seek validation from every date, conversation, and sexual experience. To be less sensitive.

What's that? You don't like the fact I enjoy the odd cigarette? Bye-bye, then.

Oh, you prefer women who aren't moms? Okay, see ya.

Hmmm? Long legs up to her ears, eh? Might I suggest the zoo?

I just needed to shift my brain into objective gear and wrap some Teflon around my heart.

Daniel *did* end up calling me again. Half a dozen times actually, over the next three days. Finally, I "reluctantly" agreed to his invitation to watch a movie at his house. My insecurity was replaced by excitement. Here was my chance to have sex with the yummiest of young men *and* begin applying Shane's lessons.

Fresh and beautified, I got in my minivan, anticipating what our night of movie-watching would hold. *Too bad his roommate is home,* I thought. I'd wanted to arrive wearing some knee-wobbling attire. But I felt good in what I was wearing: jeans, a cool belt, and a trendy, tight T-shirt. Casual but sexy.

As I started my car, I looked through the windshield at my children's darkened bedroom windows. *Everyone's snuggled safe in bed, dreaming sweet dreams. Meanwhile, look what their crazy mom is up to,* I thought, shaking my head in disapproval.

Suddenly, over the quiet hum of the minivan engine I realized I heard guitar strumming. It was coming from my speakers: Rihanna's "Good Girl Gone Bad." Smiling, I reached over and turned it up. *Live in the now, girl,* I thought, looking ahead out my windshield. *Go have some fun!*

I shifted into gear and drove off into a night full of stars and opportunities.

Two hours later, I unlocked my front door and quietly crept inside. My baby sitter, Janice, peeked around the corner in her flannel pajamas. "Hello," she whispered. "How was your night?"

"It was really fun," I whispered back, wondering if my hair was a mess (she thought I was just out with "friends"—if she only knew!). "Everybody sleeping still?"

"Yes-yes. No problems. Not a sound all night."

"Excellent. Thanks, Janice." I walked down the hall to my bedroom and quickly changed and got ready for bed. I wasn't tired. In fact, I was kind of glowing, lingering in a post-orgasmic wonderland. My body felt wonderful . . . *fulfilled.*

The health experts were right, I thought to myself with a grin. *Sex is good for our health. I guess sex doesn't have to be heart-centered to be of value. Maybe fun and physical pleasure could be meaning enough.*

I sat down at my desk and began composing my "date

report" to Shane. Overall, our evening had gone really well. But in terms of my "dominating" him, *hmm*, that was another story. Prior to ending up in his bedroom, my behavior was anything but assertive. I acted more like a demure, wholesome teenager than a confident, dominant woman. All that was missing were my braces and big Madonna bow. What I *wanted* to do was pounce on him and tear off his clothes. What I *really* did was sit beside him, watch TV for half an hour, and *wish* I was ripping off his clothes. First, we pretended we didn't notice we were touching legs. Then, we graduated to hand-holding. Then, a hand with a mind of its own got to leg rubbing. And finally, we met in the middle for a kiss.

But *mmmm*, that kiss sure melted away our awkwardness. As soon as lips made contact, we full-on attacked each other like horny teenagers on their parents' couch; cushions were either tossed or stampeded hard! And when he whispered "let's move to the bed" and stood up to whip his shirt off, I struggled to get up like a horizontal toddler in a ball pit.

My domination mission pretty much flew out of my brain and out the window. The sheer beauty of his god-like physique was one thing, but to see it and feel it ripple and flex in action was enough to send my brain into overload. My little snowboarder was ripe with style and endurance to match—and he zigzagged around my body like I was his human black diamond run (godDAMN, I could never do a ski team!). A couple of times midcourse, I did try to teach him the Chad Maneuver. But he didn't quite get it—blame it on different rhythm. But guess what? I squirted anyway! This time it happened with deep penetration while I was on top. Apparently, I have more to learn about my body than I thought.

As we removed his sheets to let the mattress dry off, I could tell he was astonished by how wet it was. "I've only been with one other girl who squirted," he revealed. "And it was a long, long time ago."

I thought, *What, were you twelve or something?* I *did* feel a tiny bit embarrassed by my mess, but on the other hand, I thought, *You better get used to it, junior!*

So, although I had a great night of sex, I didn't quite succeed in my mission. My main objective in dating younger men, other than expending some pent-up sexual energy, was to step outside the lines of my safe little boundaries and take more than just a "peek" beyond the fence. I wanted to sit in the feeling of power and see if it had anything to teach me. I wanted to be more aggressive, self-assured, demanding, risk-taking—in bed and out of bed. I wanted to verbalize what I wanted, play with his mind a bit, and stop being so self-conscious. And tonight, all the cards were perfectly lined up. In fact, I knew he *wanted* me to dominate him. *So what* if Daniel's roommate was home. I should have tossed the movie disc across the room, pushed him against the wall, kissed him hard, and *then* told him to sit in a different chair while I watched my favorite TV show—in my bra and panties. Now *that* would have caused some tension. But instead, I'd reverted to "nice girl" conduct—*urghh!* I obviously still had some pretty ingrained habits to shed; this mission would require another attempt.

I quickly hammered out a brief synopsis of my evening for Shane and added a couple happy faces at the end. No use rambling on to him about my personal revelations; those were mine, not his. At the end of my email, I added: "I'm talking to a couple of other guys too. I'll keep you posted."

Cigarette time. I threw on my winter jacket and went out the backdoor to smoke beneath the clear, starlit sky.

Shane's email awaited me in the morning:

> *Finally*, the woman had sex. Just don't wimp out on seeing the others now. The "Queen" needs to see all the

candidates. Whether you decide to have one lover or five, there is no shame in having non-lame sex. You now need to accept the responsibilities in getting what you are entitled to, including pursuing it more consciously and regularly.

My sense is that you are still being the classy, nice girl of old. You *need* to be judgmental; you *need* to actively set the terms of how any ongoing situation is set up. You are the BOSS. It is fundamentally up to YOU to decide what happens.

With that, I went after my next conquest. A week later, I was in his apartment.

Mission No. 3
Subject's name: Minotaur Brent
Age: 28
Body Type: 6 feet tall and husky
Penis Size: reported as "plenty and then some" (unconfirmed)

I quickly foresaw that Brent was going to be a harder case to break than Adonis Boy.

In our correspondence, we clearly jockeyed for the dominant role. I said he was not to kiss me without permission; he said I'd beg him to. I said I was the one in control; he said, we'll see about that. I said I'm older and will demand what I want; he said he's been with older women before. Not once did he show signs of submissiveness. Nor did our age difference seem to be fulfilling some juvenile fantasy.

I agreed to meet him spur of the moment on a Wednesday night (after the kids were in bed) at his condo. Not inside his condo, but outside, so I could assess him. I watched as he exited the main floor elevator and walked toward me. He was clean-cut, with a full head of short dark hair. He was wearing a heavy jacket so I couldn't see his physique, but he looked fit—more thickly built than Daniel.

After talking outside for about fifteen minutes, it was clear he was normal *and* that we had chemistry. Since we were darn near freezing out in the cold, I accepted his invitation to go up to his condo. He promised to behave; we'd simply chat.

We sat side by side on his couch and chatted for about half an hour while the TV played quietly in the background. I was surprised at how comfortable I felt. *You're in some guy's condo that you just met!* a voice screeched. *What if he's hiding a knife under the couch?*

Oh, hush. I smiled at myself and leaned further into the couch. I was actually really enjoying his company. His energy was strong but calm, and I found it rather sexy.

Suddenly, I realized he was staring at me with a big smirk on his face. "What?" I asked, eyebrows high. "Why are you looking at me like that?"

He chuckled. "I just can't help but notice that you're not nearly as bossy in person as you are online. You're actually really sweet. And really *hot*." And before I could cleverly respond, he pulled me down on top of him on the couch.

As his hands began roaming my back, Shane's words came back to me: "Nobody takes from you without asking. Got it?" *I hear you, Shane, but it's really hard when it feels so good! Plus, my left arm is pinned underneath him!*

Calmly, masterfully, Brent turned his head so that our lips were dangerously close. "I told you not to kiss me," I warned him. "Any kissing will be decided by me."

"I know." His dark eyes went from my eyes to my lips. "I'm not kissing you." Strong, gentle hands explored my body through the outside of my clothes. My one free arm was no match for his two stronger ones.

My body roused at his touch . . . and I realized I was caving. I had to get out of there before I went AWOL on my mission. With a sudden spurt of resolve, I yanked my pinned arm out from underneath him and jumped to my feet. "I'm *going* now, Brent," I said, brushing my disheveled clothes back into place. I marched to the door.

"It was very nice to meet you, Brent," I added, as I fumbled in the corridor to zip up my high-heeled boots. His large presence loomed beside me.

"You too, Delaine." That same smirk . . . *Grrrr.*

I pulled my jacket off the hangar and swung it over my arm. "Alrighty then," I said firmly. "I think I've got everything." I faced him directly for a split second. "I will talk to you later." I turned and walked the few steps to the door. *Just keep moving! Do NOT look back.*

Suddenly, his hand was on my arm. He pulled me around and pinned me solidly against the door. He kissed me hard, and oh my God, he was so deliciously sexy, I caved. My jacket and purse fell to the floor. He picked me up, held my legs around his waist, and carried me back down the hallway toward his bedroom.

"No Brent!" I said breathlessly, in between his determined kisses. "I'm not going to have sex with you." He quickly turned and backed me into another wall, still kissing me and gripping my legs around him. No one had ever picked me up for that long before, but he made it seem so easy. His strong legs leaned into me while his thick shoulders and back rippled with the power of a bull. *Oh my God—I was being devoured by a Minotaur!*

I'm not sure how long he held me there or how long we kissed. My head spun and my body raged with lust. Eventually, I slid to the floor, after which he grabbed me and turned me to face the wall. Again, his big hands seemed to be everywhere on my body. I had to make a decision!

I crouched down and ducked out of his reach. "'K, I'm *leaving!*"

I raced to the door, grabbing my stuff along the way, and opened it. Once safely outside in the corridor I looked back at him, breathing heavy, hair disheveled. "*Good night,* Brent," I said, unable to hide my exasperation.

He leaned in the doorway, smirking in that same infuriating but sexy way, his dark thick hair screaming to be tousled. "I'll talk to you soon, Delaine," he murmured. And his gaze warmed my back as I walked to the elevator.

Once home, I quickly shooed out the baby sitter and dove onto my computer.

> Shane:
>
> So I met with my other young man tonight. I'm so turned on right now I can't even think straight. He may be young, Shane, but I think he's a budding alpha. He refused to let me lead and picked me up and pinned me against the wall at the end of the night. I walked out on him before my clothes were off, but it took every ounce of my strength!
>
> His demeanor—and his TOUCH—wow, they made me melt, Shane! I really don't know if I have it in me to make him submit to me. I just feel the insatiable desire to have sex with him!

True to form, Shane's response was waiting in my inbox the next morning.

> *Hmmm.* I think you need to get through a mega-slutty phase before you can focus on dominating this or any man. Until your pussy is satisfied, I think domination will take a back seat.

Again, there is no shame in having great sex on your terms with as many partners as you choose. I don't want to hear any more whining about you being lonely and horny on weekends anymore. In fact, I think it might be good for you to venture even further outside your comfort zone: Why not take two different lovers on any given weekend? Just think, double the satisfaction . . .

Two lovers in one weekend? I sat there wide-eyed. No way! Hah, what kind of girl does he think I am?

Well, hold on . . . *hmmm.* I needed to think about this with a level head. Maybe, just maybe, I *could.* I was already heading down that road with Adonis Boy Daniel and Minotaur Brent. I just assumed they'd be spaced out.

My imagination shot off, my protests left coughing in the dust: me on a Friday night, greeting Adonis Boy at the door in a dynamite red dress; there'd be no silly hand-holding on the couch this time. Then me, on a Saturday night, being pinned hard against the wall by Minotaur Brett. *Mmmm* . . . those big shoulders, those strong legs. Wow. Talk about a weekend smorgasbord of sheer yumminess.

But would I feel like a slut afterward? Or would I be skipping down the street with a mischievous twinkle in my eye? I couldn't figure out which was crazier: to act on such opportunities, or *not* act on them.

That darn Shane! I growled, smiling all the same. Even though he was pushing me outside of my comfort zone, I felt compelled to do it simply to prove to him that I could.

"Are you *really* a powerful lioness, Delaine?" he seemed to taunt. "Or are you nothing but a poor little scardie' cat? I *dare* you, Delaine."

And the headstrong part of me snapped: "You just watch!" But I would never do it just for Shane. This had to be something *I* wanted; nothing less.

CHAPTER 12
OPERATION DOUBLE SATISFACTION

MORE THAN SIX MONTHS HAD passed since the Graham bomb went off—198 days to be exact—and the trees surrounding my house were almost empty of leaves. Another 176 days in the wilderness lay ahead of me before I'd hit the one-year mark, that pivotal first anniversary where my life was bound to look "way better," as Hali put it. I really did feel like I'd made progress. But then again, maybe when you've gone a little insane, you really don't care where you are.

In my mind's eye, I still saw myself trudging through the wilds, feeling lost and unsure. But periodically, I caught myself having a laugh—no, *sharing* a laugh—with someone else. It was that part of me I liked to call my "Wild Woman," an aspect of myself I'd suppressed throughout my marriage who was really doing much of the guiding in my postdivorce metamorphosis.

And not only had I gotten used to her presence, I'd grown to like her. She was energetic, fun, playful—and she egged on my more inhibited, overly cautious self. I felt like she was propelling my life forward, setting things in motion . . . though I sensed my wiser, more "mature" aspects were standing by, cringing and white-knuckled.

Now before you start thinking "multiple personality

disorder," let me explain. I believe that women have different aspects or sides of themselves. Kind of like wearing different "hats." And each of these "aspects" of me came with a set of her own distinct qualities—strengths and weaknesses—that together served a specific purpose. Collectively, they represented the expansiveness of my soul.

I'm sure behavioral scientists and academics have a fancy term for the layers of our personalities, but to me, they were like a series of inner-Delaines, all slightly different in character. And I liked to name mine: Wise Woman, Little Girl, Mother Soul, Warrior Woman, Wild Woman, and so on. I pictured these aspects sitting on a committee together, and as life situations arose, each one took a turn sharing her opinion about the matter at hand. For the past seven years, the head chairperson had been my Mother Soul. Her voice and opinion carried the most weight. But when the Graham bomb exploded, I think the boardroom flew into a state of chaos and mutiny. Low and behold, I believe a new leader mongered her way into the chairperson's seat: Wild Woman.

But because I was still getting to know this side of me, I was wary of her judgment. Maybe I should be ignoring her or throwing rocks at her. Maybe she was trouble in disguise and luring me to the dreaded "Dark Side." *Hmmm. Would that make Shane my Darth Vader?*

But my instincts said she didn't mean me any harm. In fact, it felt more like she was trying to help me, teach me. Maybe even remind me or reconnect me with a part of myself I once knew.

My sense was that she wasn't going to hold onto her "seat" for too long though. Other committee members wanted to throttle her! Nonetheless, not only did she make good company in the "wilderness" I was currently slogging through, she seemed to know these parts; I was in *her* territory. And my gut said she might be the one to guide me out of here.

I SWEAR I did *not* set out to do it intentionally, despite Shane's challenge. I swear it was more by chance than deliberate effort. But yes, only two weeks after the challenge was issued, I had sex with two different men during one weekend! To my credit, it was a long weekend, with a forty-eight-hour gap between lovers instead of twenty-four. Still, it counts in *my* rule book.

I was positively beaming as I emailed my accomplishment to Shane. Feeling feisty, I tacked onto the end: "It's raining men. And I do, in fact, feel like a 'QUEEN.' Maybe you're right— maybe I *am* a slut after all! (Meaning only a woman who loves to orgasm, of course.)"

Surprise-surprise, one of my lovers turned out to be Football Coach Chad (he was no longer a stupid jock). And the other was Minotaur Brent; let's just say I had "pressing," unfinished business with him.

On Friday night, the Minotaur and I picked up where we'd left off; that is, I was wrapped around his waist and pinned against the wall. This time I didn't fight the rippling beast. Actually, that's not true. I *did* fight him—by "resisting" him and acting nonchalant. But he easily saw through my pretense; he knew I wanted him to win. So he carefully tested my "no's," pushing them a little further, then a little further. "You're a bad girl, Delaine," he whispered in my ear. "You know you want my hard cock between your legs. *Say* it."

To which I'd respond, "The only one in desperate need right now is you, young man." Eventually, he had my hands held tight against my back, his obvious hardness pressed against my stomach.

My involuntary moans made my true desires transparent.

His force aroused me. It wouldn't have used to. The Delaine I'd always known enjoyed gentle caresses, sensual touches, a look-me-deep-in-the-eyes kind of intimacy. Yet suddenly, it seemed I yearned to be taken, filled, physically overpowered if need be. Not just by any man, of course. *But one who I deemed worthy.* My match. My equal. Not of souls. But of mind and body only. It was pure carnal desire gone ballistic, or maybe just a simple case of hormones. Whatever the case, despite what I soon discovered was a noticeably smaller-than-average penis, I G-spot orgasmed numerous times—and *squirted. Small, shmall.* I wasn't grumbling too much about penis size. Maybe it really *was* the motion of the ocean and not the size of the ship.

However, his *reaction* to my squirting didn't impress me.

"Did you *pee?*" he asked, startled. He even looked a little disgusted.

"*What?* No!" I said, taken aback. "I climaxed. And when I orgasm I sometimes release a clear liquid. Lots of it. I *squirt.*"

"Oh," he replied lamely. "I thought you peed the bed."

Duh! "It's something I started doing not too long ago. I take it you've never been with a girl who squirts?"

"Nope." His voice was so monotone it irritated me. Perhaps I was hoping he'd be impressed? Apparently, it's not a turn-on for every man. *Pfft*, couldn't he at least show some interest?

Despite his ambivalence, I did not feel ashamed or embarrassed about my body—which was a big shift for me. (Hit the applause button.) In the past, I would have been ashamed if a man was put off by my body in any way. (Score one for the team!). If the Minotaur had a problem with me leaving a puddle when I orgasmed, well then, he could go back to the enchanted forest and track down a virgin princess.

Despite the uneven end to our evening, my clash with the Minotaur reinforced something powerful and new about myself: that my body's ability to experience the intense pleasure of G-spot orgasm was *not* contingent on one or two men's sexual prowess. My marvelous new talent was all mine to pack up, take with me, and enjoy with whomever I wanted.

Feeling inspired, I spent the next day and a half attacking a household project that I'd put off for months (alright, *years*): I painted my daughter's bedroom. Goodbye star stencils, hello sunshine yellow! While on a roll, I also sorted through her closets and drawers, bagging up old and outgrown clothes for the Good Will. I viewed the results of my hard work with a smile: Now *this* was satisfying!

Then, out of the blue, Chad called. Yup, talk about unexpected. He apologized profusely, citing football games and practices as reasons for his disappearance. I decided to let him off the hook—not because I fully believed him but because my body wanted to see him.

I didn't think his poor behavior warranted a sexy "Delaine-o-Gram" entrance, so I showed up wearing a stylish pink T and jeans, toting an overnight bag stuffed with my Super Girl jammies. And as we sat on his couch, feeling relaxed, our conversation flowing easily, I inwardly grinned at his feature wall painting: some NHL goalie making a save. *Such a jock. And obviously a bachelor!*

Suddenly, he was leaning into me on the couch. His lips were on my neck, sending warmth throughout my stomach. "So . . ." he said softly, as I sat there, eyes closed. "I covered my bed with a plastic parachute."

I burst out laughing. "What?"

He stood up and added playfully: "*And* four layers of towels—actually, I think I emptied most of my linen closet. And I've got scuba gear beside the bed, you know—just in case."

I laughed harder, "Maybe move the water cooler in there too so I don't get dehydrated."

"Done!" he said, as he pulled me to my feet and into his chest. More seriously: "Now let's go see how many times I can make you squirt."

An offer I couldn't refuse.

Suffice it to say, our time together was amazing; the same as it was our first time together only longer and more intense. We changed the sheets twice.

This time when we said goodbye, I commanded him sweetly not to wait so long to phone. Our sexual chemistry was so dynamite, I felt confident he'd follow my orders.

So not only did I experience two nights of passion with two different men, I also completed Shane's assigned mission. I had to rate Operation Double Satisfaction a hands-down success.

The Duke and his games aside, personally I felt completely at peace with my actions; no regrets. No guilt. Moreover, I felt *proud of myself.* I stepped outside my boundaries and experienced something new that felt empowering and didn't hurt anyone. I allowed myself to be a little wild and be a little "bad" (if only in the context of "conventional" mores), and it was incredibly fun, sexy, and satisfying. I'd had a Super Girl weekend, that's for sure. That said, I didn't plan to broadcast it around, even to my more open-minded friends. Just Hali, as always. Besides, I soon learned she had her own story to tell. And she actually outscored me. *The vixen!*

After their heated email repartee reached the breaking point, Hali finally met up with the Mini Val Kilmer (a.k.a., "the bed-post-notcher") on Thursday, the night before I "peed" on Mino-taur Brent. Then on Saturday, she had a surprise quickie with the well-endowed Josh; and on Sunday it was with her soon-to-be ex-husband, Paul.

I was totally taken aback by the last one.

"Oh *no,* Hali—*Paul?* How did this happen?" I asked her the next morning.

"I know I know. It wasn't planned at all, Delaine. He came to my place to drop off the kids and stuck around to help me put them to bed. Afterward, he asked if he could have a glass of wine. I was in the mood for one too, so I said, 'Sure, go ahead.' Of course, we ended up finishing the bottle.

"As we talked on the couch, he started rubbing my back and running his hand through my hair. I knew where it was leading and I kept looking at the clock thinking, 'I had sex with Josh less than twenty-four hours ago. I should at least try to stall.' *(Laugh)* But, oh well. It felt right so we went upstairs and had sex."

"And how was it? Or more importantly, how do you feel now?"

There was a pause. "It was good," she said. "It was familiar, you know? He was very passionate. I think it meant a lot to him and he kept telling me how beautiful I was. But for me it was more just the physical enjoyment of sex. I'm not reading into it, Delaine. It's common for couples who break up to fall into bed a few times afterward. That's all it was."

I wasn't convinced. My sense was that he was trying to maneuver his way back into her life and I feared her vulnerability. But she sounded okay with what transpired. In fact, she seemed stuck on the fact she'd had sex with three different men in four days: "I just can't believe I had to kill time before sleeping with Paul so I could hit the twenty-four-hour mark. How bad is *that*?"

Later that night, I laid in bed grinning over our weekend's sexual escapades. Who'd have thought that the two of us were capable of such naughtiness? Somehow, knowing my best friend had been as mischievous as me made it all the more sweet. And unlike me, Hali hadn't needed a coach like Shane to dare her to do it. She simply "owned" it. Guess *her* Wild Woman just told her other committee members to shut up.

The next morning, I got mail from Shane:

Of course you're a slut. I see it every time I look at your coy little photos. I'm glad you enjoyed yourself last weekend and feel good about it. You see, this is the stuff I like. I enjoy effecting a woman's actions even when miles away. The orgasms you had were partly caused by me. Admit it: you orgasmed partly because of me, didn't you? Think about that. Maybe you should think about thanking me for helping you have your best orgasms ever. Maybe you should think about how your sexuality took a quantum leap forward just from having a taste of me and how it might improve more dramatically if you give yourself to me more.

I sat there with my mouth agape. I guess I had been expecting a jubilant high-five, not . . . *this*. It felt like a half-reprimand, half-reminder that my weekend men were but puny sprouts compared to the "Super Alpha Man." *Grrrr,* not only was he trying to put me in "my place" again, he was titillating me with an even greater challenge: squaring off with him.

He was right, though: my actions and orgasms were, in part, because of him. Perhaps I did owe him a smidgen of gratitude. And yes, I wondered what might happen if I *did* give more of myself to him?

But I was getting ahead of myself. Because Wild Woman or not, this Super Girl could only take on so many challenges at once.

CHAPTER 13

HIDDEN DESIRES AND HOPEFULNESS

THE SCHOOL GYMNASIUM WAS PACKED full of parents when I arrived to watch my middle son, Evan's, autumn kindergarten performance. I was standing to the side, scanning the room for an empty chair, when a hand waving from the back caught my attention. It was one of my mom-friends, Tina, gesturing me over.

"We saved you a seat," she said as I sat down next to her and her husband.

"Thanks guys. I meant to come a few minutes earlier but homework was a *war* tonight, and I had to get the kids settled with my sitter."

She smiled knowingly. "We have those nights too." The lights in the room suddenly dimmed. "Good timing," she whispered.

"Ladies and gentlemen, friends and parents," the school principal announced over the microphone from center stage. "Welcome to this year's kindergarten performance of *Songs from Around the World*."

The room was abuzz with parent anticipation. Actually, this was an all-out family affair: younger siblings climbing in their seats, moms and dads perched side by side with video cameras, a grandparent or two reclining and browsing through the program. I noticed that a lot of fathers were present, some in their work suits, a few sitting alone. Though I had attended countless past events solo when Robert was out of town, tonight I felt my "singleness" acutely amid all these families. I wondered: *How many of these men are separated or divorced?*

All at once, music boomed over the loudspeakers and children paraded onto the stage and through the gym's side doors. The room exploded with their sweet voices, a sound so angelic it brought tears to my eyes. I searched through the hoards of children smartly dressed in their navy blue and white uniforms, until there, off on the right side of the stage, I saw my son's wild red hair. His mouth was moving, but I could tell he was looking for me. I half-stood and waved, again . . . and again . . . until finally our eyes met. He waved back immediately, beaming from ear-to-ear. I nodded enthusiastically: *Don't worry, Mommy's here!* And he carried on singing, now more animatedly.

The opening number ended with mighty applause. Cameras flashed like paparazzi. As tiny feet scurried off the stage, I quickly scanned the program. His class wasn't performing until the last act. That meant five other kindergarten classes to sit through. *Sigh.*

As the first act commenced (some ditty about China), my attention shifted. There, in the back of the dark, elementary school auditorium, buried amid row after row of seemingly devoted moms and dads, my mind floated to a wholly different realm.

The tape rolled, unedited snippets of X-rated footage from last weekend's sexual encounters: The Minotaur then Chad, Chad then The Minotaur. *Hungry lips on my skin, a rough hand caressing my nipple, hard muscles engaged, groans from the throat, strong hands clenching my hips . . .* Could I even tell them apart in my reverie? It was all just sizzling touches and erotic captions relived, replayed, over and over and over.

I felt a sudden warm rush. My body responded in the here and now. I sat up tall in my seat and crossed my legs. *Welcome back.*

Did anyone notice I was gone? Am I looking in the right direction? Oh, everyone's laughing. Smile along, look engaged.

Man, this is so bad, I thought, feeling *really* guilty. *Instead of marveling at my son's first kindergarten performance, I'm off in a sexual fantasy world!*

I gazed at the faces and profiles of those near me. I was looking for evidence, signs, clues about their *real* lives: secret passions, hidden desires. I wondered who had a fulfilling sex life, a passionate lover in the wings, or maybe no sex at all. Surely I couldn't be the only one with something to hide.

Suddenly, a man in the row ahead looked back over his shoulder at me. We locked eyes for a long second until I pulled mine away. What made him turn away from the stage? Did he unconsciously feel my wanton sexual energy? Did he see "Wild Divorcee" written all over me? Please don't let his wife look back, too. She'll *know.* She'll know I'm a "promiscuous girl." I swear I'm transparent.

Oh my God, I am so paranoid. I just can't seem to escape it. Might as well go ahead and write in on my tombstone:

LOVING MOM, DEDICATED FRIEND,
HAD SEX WITH TWO DIFFERENT MEN IN ONE WEEKEND.
DEVOTED HER LIFE TO WORRYING ABOUT IT.

But now that I'd had a few days to digest last weekend's promiscuity, my mind was at war with itself *and* my body. Why the heck did I call it "promiscuity" anyway? I hated that word. It was so judgmental and, well, *limiting.* Why couldn't I think of it as "sexual exploration"? Yes, that sounded way more empowering.

Where had this shrill, paranoid voice inside my head come from? Was it high school? *Man, I perseverate!* I thought back twenty-three years to that crazy self-defining time when I heard whispered rumors about "so and so" being a slut. Talk was vicious and spread like wildfire. No one had a clue how to keep a secret at that age, and once a girl was labeled, she was marked for good.

High school may have acted as a launch pad for my beliefs, but they were most certainly reinforced and drilled home afterward. In university, the workplace, the neighborhood, bars, sometimes even family gatherings, talk about "some woman" was bound to get cheap. It still did.

I'd naively assumed that the popularity of TV shows like *Sex in the City* and *Desperate Housewives* indicated that times had changed, that women could be seen as respectable and moral *and* sexual beings. But on closer look, that's really wasn't the case at all, was it? We still held our breaths when our favorite characters fell into bed with yet *another* man. They could only make so many mistakes. We still judged their actions: warranted? Or inexcusably whorish?

Then, there were the full-blown slut characters that we loved to hate. Look at Super Slut Samantha Jones who unapologetically "has sex like a man." Carrie and the gang were ahead of the rest of us, accepting and loving and valuing her despite *and* because of her sexual lifestyle. But how many women would have frowned and whispered behind her back as soon as she left the table? Or even invited her to lunch in the first place?

And because I'm not just a woman, but a Divorced Mom, the harsh judgments potentially cast my way scared me to death. After all, "decent" divorced mothers should never engage in casual sex, right? Otherwise these women were loose, irresponsible, unfit mothers: the stereotype "divorcee." That's right; the insidious "D" word. Better lock up your husbands, ladies. No—decent divorced mothers should only want a serious relationship. And they better get on that quick, because with each year that passed, they were apt to grow more bitter and undesirable and desperate. They were women with cargo. Women who'd failed. Women who didn't deserve any better. *Spit.*

I'm not even sure where my own judgments and those of society began and ended. All I knew was that I never dreamed of waking up at this point in my life a single mother of three. But reality dose: Here I was! And contrary to what any rule books may say, I knew beyond any morsel of doubt that I was not "dried up" and dead! Why couldn't society trust me to be a good mother (amongst many other things), *and* allow me to be in charge of my own sexuality? Why should my "adventures," which were helping me to heal, grow, and transform during a radical period of change, be a source of embarrassment or shame?

"We have to be careful about who we discuss our dating lives with," Hali had warned me a month back. "You and I want to talk about this stuff because it's exciting and scary and we're suddenly single again. And we naturally assume that the people we love will understand us. But the truth is, most people can't relate to it."

Her warning had come after a conversation she'd had with her close, longtime friend Megan over lunch one day. Hali, accustomed to being open and honest with her, was rambling on about a twenty-nine-year-old man she'd met at a bar. The more she talked, the more she became aware of the disapproval in her friend's eyes. When she'd confronted Megan about it, her friend replied defensively, "But I'm not judging you! You know I love you."

"Yes you are!" Hali responded. "I can see it in your eyes! We all filter information through our own experiences and then judge it. And you are a dear friend who has three kids and has been happily married for fifteen years and you are looking at and judging my situation through your set of glasses! I can *feel* it."

Ultimately, her friend agreed to disagree, and conversation around dating was indefinitely shut down.

I heeded Hali's warning, but I already knew to restrict who I told of my escapades. Remember—I'd felt my own pangs of caution during the summer when I'd met with my "mom-friends" at the local pub. They were so curious about what single life looked like for a woman of our age. But my intuition kept telling me to be cautious; they *were* judging me, consciously or not.

It's the difference between not having kids but having an *opinion* about motherhood. Having wild sex with multiple partners after separation wasn't a pair of shoes most had walked in, and sexual promiscuity was a contentious zone to begin with; it could be hot and juicy yet still trigger judgment, even moral outrage. Even if the listener was a lovely friend—a strong, mature, independent mother and career woman—her ethical boundaries around sex could be rigid and unforgiving. And I didn't want to be the next candidate up for a stoning.

I thought about my three-year-old daughter and what I hoped for her to experience some day, within her own sexuality. In terms of her partner "numbers," my knee-jerk reaction was to say, "Make sure you can count them on two hands!" But my response came from fear: fear of her being judged and shunned by others, and fear that her choices would come from a place of unworthiness instead of empowerment. Big difference.

What I *really* hoped was that her heart wouldn't be broken too much, that she would find deep, meaningful love and/or friendship in a relationship (or three or ten), and that she would live a passionate, fulfilling life. As for her numbers, I wanted her to be able to make that decision 100 percent on her own terms. No one else's.

I now realized that every single sexual partner I'd had thus far had taught me something—about him, about sex, about our relationship, and about me. Bad or good, my Self was expanding, and each liaison had opened new levels of awareness. I wanted that freedom of self for my daughter as well. I wanted her to feel whole and fulfilled, not through self-denial and adherence to some societal code, but through her own conscious choices. I wanted her to sit strongly in her body, to listen to it and trust it; to understand that her sexuality was one of *many* vital aspects of who she was, and that she was entitled to explore it—however she saw fit. And if she made numerous mistakes along her journey, I hoped she would learn from them, then *keep on going* instead of wallowing in feelings of regret or shame.

ACT SIX OPENED with the sounds of banjoes and fiddles filling the gymnasium. Hand-in-hand, two children at a time ventured forth on stage into a fluid circular formation. And here came my son! I joined in with the other parents who were clapping along to the barnyard beat. *Wow, look at him dance! He's quite the performer, my boy.*

At the end of the song, he looked directly at me. BIG smile. *He's so gorgeous!* I vigorously clapped and gave him a standing ovation. Suddenly, I felt tears in my eyes. *Gosh, I'm such a mom.* But I can't help it. Whenever I look at him, or any of my children, I see white light. They shine and display their loving faith in the world with such ease and brilliance.

With tightness in my chest, I continued clapping. Silently, I prayed that no man or woman would stomp out my children's light—*that* would be the greatest and cruelest sin in my book. Especially my daughter. I knew what she'd be up against. Above all, I wished her the freedom to cultivate and share her marvelous "whole" authentic self with this vast and complicated world.

CHAPTER 14

THE LIONESS MUST DEVOUR THE DIK-DIK

Mission No. 4
Subject's Name: Black Cloud Brian
Age: 43
Body Type: tall, fit, really nice bum
Penis Size: undisclosed, but hoping for plenteous

ALTHOUGH I WAS OFFICIALLY OUT on "assignment" for this date, secretly I hoped it might he more. I'd already met Brian for coffee a few days earlier, and I was pleasantly thrilled by what walked through the door: Mr. Tall and Handsome with a motorcycle helmet under his arm. Not only was this guy really smart, he was also incredibly funny. I nearly spit out my drink from laughing so hard. Turns out, he was a professional comedian. And at the end of our first date, as he strode off to the men's bathroom, I observed from tableside that his butt looked lovely in his jeans and black leather chaps.

For this second date, he'd invited me and a couple of my friends to the comedy club where he was the emcee. I had dressed with an after-hour rendezvous in mind: a fitted black dress with spaghetti straps that concealed a black, lacy bustier and garters. Oh, and of course: fishnet stockings and black high-heeled boots.

In addition to Hali, our friend Tara, who was in town visiting, was also joining me. She, too, was struggling with an abusive philanderer of a husband and had moved to the West Coast a year ago to be closer to her extended family *and* make a final decision about her comatose marriage. Now pushing forty, she'd been married to him (a former professional athlete) since she was twenty-four. She'd poured her heart into their relationship and two children, despite his affair, despite his anger issues and physical abuse, despite his feeble communication skills, and *even* despite his complete sexual disinterest in her.

For years, I'd listened to Tara grapple aloud about her unfulfilling sex life. Whether she dressed up in lace, warmed him up with a relaxing massage, or backed away from him entirely, he never initiated sex and rarely played along. She analyzed their sex life over and over again: Was her wanting it more than once a month too much? Shouldn't she just accept the fact that his libido was lower than hers? Shouldn't she focus on feeling grateful for other, more positive aspects of their marriage? Because that's what she'd tried to do: count her blessings and love him for the other ways he gave to her and the kids. But inevitably, she ended up feeling like she was *convincing* herself she was happy. Wasn't that the same thing as "settling"? One thing was blatantly clear: His consistent disinterest in her was hurting her. Struggle as she did to accept it, his indifference translated into "You aren't desirable—as a partner *or* a woman."

Tonight, as we indulged in a few greasy appetizers and a liter of wine, Tara brought us up to speed on her West Coast life. And the more I listened to her talk, the more my stomach knotted with empathy. I saw my old self as I looked at her, this long-haired, stylishly dressed woman with *sad blue eyes*. She was clinging onto the scraps of kindness and physical affection he sporadically threw her, telling herself it was enough to subsist on. Her family was her dream, and she was resolute about enduring whatever life had to throw at them. As she put it, her marriage "hadn't become bad *enough* to leave." Hali and I listened with compassion, love, and support, knowing that only she could make any final decision.

As the conversation switched to mine and Hali's lives, the mood suddenly became much lighter. *And* mischievous. Because remember, up to this point, Hali and I had kept our goings-on mainly between us—we knew our crazy dating/sex stories could be easily misjudged by others. But Tara was a most trusted and welcome exception.

In the midst of our laughter over some intimate detail or another, Hali's cell phone suddenly bleeped. She held it open over the table and shook her head. "I just got a text message from Josh. He wrote, 'Can I come over for coffee?' But look how he spelled coffee—" She held out her phone and we leaned in to read it: "cofie."

"Who the hell doesn't know how to spell coffee?" she exclaimed. "Honestly, he is the worst speller ever. Yesterday he sent me a text and wrote good morning. Not 'morning,' as normal, smart people spell it, but as in someone just died: m-o-u-r-ning."

We burst out laughing, drawing curious—dare I say even envious—looks from the table beside us.

"Now which guy is this?" Tara asked. "Back up here, because I get your men confused."

"Josh is the young guy with the really big penis," Hali stated matter-of-factly. "I met him by accident when I was supposed to meet another guy on a date."

"Oh yes," said Tara nodding, as if we were discussing an education issue around our kids. "And what's he like? Besides his big penis, I mean."

"Well . . ." began Hali, leaning back in her chair and looking at me. I was already holding in giggles. "He's *not* very smart, as his text messages clearly show. He has *no* money, and he can't hold down a job. Actually, he just got fired from his construction job on the weekend for telling his boss to fuck off. Ummm, what else . . . We fight all the time. And he's *not* good-looking at all."

"He's not?" Tara was bewildered. "I was thinking he must be really hot to compensate! What does he look like?"

"Well . . . " Hali began again, a huge grin on her face. I bit my lip. "He's not very tall. Maybe five-foot-seven. His face is okay, I guess. He has skinny arms . . . a big belly . . . okay teeth, I guess."

Tara's eyes were enormous. "So *why* are you seeing this guy? I must not be getting something." She looked at me, then back at Hali.

"Honestly Tara, *it's because he has an enormous cock.*" I couldn't hold in my giggles anymore. Though I already knew Hali's story, listening to my gorgeous, *usually* classy girlfriend tell it made it all the more hilarious.

Hali continued, attempting to look serious. "There is absolutely no other reason, Tara. We have phenomenal sex and he makes me orgasm like crazy. Plus—" Hali paused. "I guess I shouldn't say it's the *only* reason. He also makes me feel great about my body. He has so many imperfections that I'm not as self-conscious about my baby weight."

"Hali," replied Tara, leaning in. "You really need to wake up and realize that you and your beautiful curves are pretty much every man's dream come true. And God—" She gestured at Hali's ripe chest. "Look at those fucking boobs!" We laughed.

"But back to his big penis," Tara continued. "As I see it, a girl has her needs and they should be taken care of; it's great he can satisfy you in that way. So tell me, have you introduced him to any of your friends?"

"No way!" Hali declared vehemently. "Not even Delaine has met him." Tara looked at me and I shook my head.

"But we do go out for lunch and shopping sometimes,"

explained Hali. "The problem is that he doesn't have a car. So I always have to go pick him up and drop him off."

By now, I was straining hard to keep my composure. I mean, "Auntie Hali" picking up and dropping off her dependant, delinquent lover? They were a walking oxymoron, and I never, in a hundred years, would have imagined her dating (or having the patience) for a goofball like this! I was laughing so hard, I had to wipe away tears.

"Tell her what happened the one time you went out to the Red Robin restaurant," I finally managed to squeak out.

"Oh yeah," said Hali, nodding. "*And* he curses a lot and has no manners. We went out for lunch one day—" She glanced at me and added: "A lunch *I* had to pay for, by the way. We're sitting there in this family restaurant, there are young kids at tables all around us, when suddenly he says something and drops the "C" word three times in one sentence! He said it *loud*, too. I was totally shocked; I wanted to crawl under the table. I have no doubt that people heard him."

"Hopefully they couldn't understand him," I offered between laughs.

"No, they *would* have heard him. He might be hard to understand, but certain words come out of his mouth crystal clear, like the 'C' word."

Tara was confused. "Does he have a speech impediment, too?"

"No no," said Hali laughing. "He's got an accent. He's from Newfoundland. And his accent is *really* thick." Hali looked at me again and pushed out, between giggles, "I can't even understand what he says most of the time. *We can hardly even COMMUNICATE!*" And with that, Hali roared with laughter too. She added, "*Why* am I with this guy? Oh my, I really must be *desperate*." That was it; all three of us were in tears now.

Two minutes later, just as we started to compose ourselves,

a deep lively voice boomed over the microphone: "Good evening, everyone! How are y'all doing tonight?" The crowd cheered. I smiled; I'd almost forgotten why I was here.

"Is that *him?*" Tara whispered, her eyes glued to the long-legged man on stage wearing blue jeans and a Budweiser T-shirt.

"Yeah," I whispered back.

"He's hot."

And very funny, too, as it turned out. I'm not sure if it was entirely his talent or my giddy mood from Josh stories that made me laugh so much. But by the end of the evening, my jaw muscles and cheeks were aching.

As the club began to clear out, Hali, Tara, and I lingered at our table to finish our last sips of wine. "Go over and talk to him," urged Tara.

"Nah," I responded. "He knows I'm here. He'll come over when he's ready."

"And here he comes *now,*" said Hali, on high alert. All three of us got to our feet as he approached the table. Hali and Tara started putting on their coats.

"Hey ladies," he said casually, while staring at me from head to toe. "You heading home already?"

"*We* are," said Hali, gesturing to Tara. "But *she's* free." She poked me in the side.

"Would you like to grab a drink next door?"

"Sure," I said. I turned and hugged my girlfriends.

"Have fun," whispered Tara with a giggle. "But play carefully."

Goes without saying, I thought, giving her a big squeeze.

Goodbyes done, Brian and I stood facing each other: a tall, bright-eyed comedian, and an equally bright-eyed babe wearing garters, each of us thinking the same thing. Let's get *this* show on the road.

GRAVITY WAS FAST in motion and there was no stopping it. Halfway through my steaming cup of tea, I actually wished Brian's mouth would stop moving. Where did the funny, confident man from my first date go? The one I just saw on stage? I sat there shell-shocked as *this* guy lamented about his ex-wife and past girlfriend, both of whom thought he was a dead-beat dad and loser: "They never understood my need to chase my dream, you know? Sure, life as a comedian is tough and the pay sucks, but it's what I wanted to do. As soon as I got rid of them, I sold my car, bought a Harley, and started going on tour."

Now, I'm all for dream chasers, so I perked up and threw him an easy shot at deliverance: "Being on tour must be exciting; traveling to new cities, meeting new people, standing in the spotlight . . ."

"No. It's not glamorous at all. I'm only doing small venues in hick towns across the prairies. And I'll tell you, it gets really damn cold this time of year on my Harley."

In my mind's eye, I caricatured him cruising down the highway with a scowl on his face, a black cloud floating above him, pelting him with rain. Behind him, his female demons chased him, screaming.

He continued: "Most of the time I don't have money for hotels, so I try to crash at another comedian's house. Even when I'm here in town, I can only afford a dingy basement apartment in some lady's house. Actually, I have a comedian friend crashing there tonight on the couch."

I nodded my head slowly in response. *So to top things off, you live like a student in a basement. Hmmm. Well then . . .*

"I have to use the ladies room." I excused myself and walked down the hallway purposefully: I had to get away from him.

I leaned over the bathroom sink and shook my head. What the hell was going on here? He wasn't an alpha male, he was an alpha whiner! I really just wanted to leave. *Ohhh, but I couldn't. That would be so mean.*

Well, since sex was out of the question, I might as well get back to my "assignment." Maybe if I steered conversation down a sexier, less gloomy path, he'd revert back to his former, chipper personality . . . ?

I catwalked back to the table with fresh lip gloss and a fresh attitude. That glimmer was now in my eyes. I deliberately positioned my chair so he could see my body and I oh-so-demurely lifted my skirt a tad, to show off a bit of thigh. "So, do you like my fishnet stockings?" I asked. *C'mon buddy, let's see what you're made of.*

He reached over and pinched a piece of netting. "Yeah. I haven't seen tights like those since the eighties." Cute answer, but his eyes glinted with insecurity.

"Actually," I began. "These aren't even tights—they're *stockings*. I have them attached up here to my garter belt." I lifted my skirt ever-so-slightly so he could catch a glimpse of a clasp.

And that's when Comedian Man went to J-E-L-L-O. I folded my arms and leaned forward on the table looking him straight in the eyes—unyielding, bold, *powerful*. His eyes dilated. He twitched. He sweated. Without even trying, I stared him down. *My God*, I thought, *this date is the biggest joke of the night!* I couldn't get out of there quick enough.

Very soon after, I was back home in my bedroom taking off my sexy clothes—*alone*, of course. Five minutes later, I was clean-faced and sporting my Super Girl jammies. I kicked my lingerie drawer closed with a *thud*.

Down in my office in front of my computer, I brewed over the night's events. Alpha Whiner's black cloud had followed *me* home. I hastily typed a short message to Shane: "I'm not even sure this guy had any vertebrae. I won without even trying. Get out the rejection stamp. I don't want to see this file in my face again."

The next morning, I walked to my computer knowing that Shane's reply would be there.

You are now at a place where the lioness catches the little "dik-diks": http://wikipedia.org/wiki/Dik-dik (check it). But instead of devouring them, you let them go. You need to get your blood lust up to make use of the rejected ones. Winning isn't enough. A lioness can always "win" with a dik-dik. You have to kill them, totally dominate them. That is the whole point in why the lioness hunts them.

Dik-dik? I didn't know what they were, but with a name like *that* . . .

I clicked on the link. "A small antelope that lives in the African brush . . . named for the sound it makes when alarmed . . . they stand approx 35 cm at the shoulder and weigh about 5 kg . . ." To the right of the page was a photo of an animal that looked like a cross between a midget antelope and a scrawny Bambi.

I grinned: So *this* is how Shane views submissive men; a totally demeaning, yet creative analogy nonetheless.

But do I buy it? Do I want to "devour" these creatures, my sweet little dik-dik men? Do I want to "keep them in their place" by making them do my laundry or jumping to serve my every whim and mood? Or do I want them hanging around at all?

Sigh. I really couldn't see getting any pleasure from it. And looking at the dik-dik photo, the mother in me just wanted to singsong, "*awwww*" and send him back to his own momma.

CHAPTER 15

PONYTAILED MOM VS. AUDACIOUS ONLINE DIVA

ANOTHER WEEKEND ALONE WITH my kids had passed. And it had felt *so* long. Not because of activity overload or anything particularly strenuous. It was all because of me. My tank was bone dry. Cracked.

Just after six o'clock that evening, kids fed and in the bathtub, I snuck out the backdoor for a cigarette and some quiet. Through the small bathroom window above me, I could hear the kids' voices as they played happily in the bubble-filled tub. *PLEASE don't fight for five minutes,* I thought, feeling exhausted. *Please just give me a few uninterrupted minutes to myself.*

Suddenly, guilt engulfed me. I knew damn well that if I didn't stay up so late talking to strange men online, I'd have more energy for my kids. *You need to get your priorities straight, Girl,* a disgusted voice scolded.

I inhaled deeply, lifting my hands as if in surrender to an empty backyard. Truth was, I had no defense. Triple shame on me. *But*—I thought, as I exhaled long. *I'm doing the best I can.*

I felt like I was living two separate lives: ponytailed stay-at-home mom and audacious online diva. The e-dating world continued to seduce and distract me. Like an addiction. Like an unfaithful red hot lover who I *knew* could only spell bad news.

Last night, on the Sugar Daddy site, a married man wrote that he was coming to Calgary on business. He wanted to meet me. After a quick read of his written profile, I politely, yet firmly replied that I don't date married men.

"I will give you one thousand dollars," he responded.

WHAT? "I'm not a prostitute, thank-you-very-much," I replied angrily. "And I don't date married men, regardless of wallet-size." "Two thousand."

"I'm NOT a prostitute," I pounded on my keyboard. "I'm sure you'll find other takers in Calgary if you look around."

A final email: "Five thousand dollars." And his picture was attached.

I sat there with my mouth open—both at the amount he was offering and his audacity. I clicked on the photo and looked straight into the olive-skinned face of a dark-haired man wearing an obviously expensive suit. "Who *are* you?" I asked the picture, wondering at his life story. I felt intrigued, yet disgusted and sorry for him all at the same time. I blocked him.

Last night, I also had an appalling phone conversation with a another man: some fifty-year-old oil tycoon from Texas. Although he was highly intelligent and well spoken, my spider senses started tingling when he began referring to the "nobles" (such as himself) and the "peasants" (anyone outside his social circle). He also kept asking me about my family history—diseases, genetics, if my family was well educated, etcetera. Finally, I came right out and asked what his true intentions were. His goal, he said, was to find and impregnate several women of good "breeding stock" from either Canada or the United States. Once the babies were born, he would pay off the moms while he raised the children with his immediate family.

"You've GOT to be joking," I declared.

"I'm dead serious," he said. "One twenty-five-year-old in L.A. is already three months along. I just need to find two more." He laughed.

And I hung up.

During the past couple of months, I'd received other strange requests and offers. Like a two-week vacation to an exclusive hedonistic resort. Or other impromptu trips to cities dotted all over the United States and the Caribbean. One man was specifically looking for a woman who enjoyed wearing a strap-on. He stated this in his first email to me. Another man wanted me to join him and his wife for some "honky-tonk" on their ranch. And when I told him I wasn't into women, he tried to entice me with naked photos—of HER.

What are you looking for, Delaine? I kept asking myself. I wasn't free to travel; I wasn't interested in any of these kinks. What did I *want*?

But I had no answer. My mind and heart were all over the map—and the men I was attracting proved this. The universe was responding to my overblown, under-settled, major-confused energy.

Relax! a voice would call to me in my brain. *You're simply in exploration mode. You're "doing research," so-to-speak. Like Shane said, this isn't a fortune cookie, it's a process. Over time, you'll zoom in on what you really want.*

"Moooooom!" My daughter's voice sliced through my diffuse awareness. I raced inside to help her out of the tub and dress her in her jammies for bed. Twenty minutes later, all three kids sat on the family room couch, gobbling up chopped fruit, while I threw on Walt Disney's *Pocahontas*.

Normally, I was a Nazi-police when it came to controlling TV and movie-watching time. But tonight, I ached for some dead-brain time. A movie was the perfect way to be with the kids in body, if not in mind and heart.

But I'd forgotten: children have no movie-watching etiquette. Their questions started flying:

"Are Indians *real* mom?"

"Why is their hair sticking up?"

"This show is TRUE? Is Pocahontas here *now?*

Finally, I blurted: "Just watch the movie guys! You're missing it!"

As if on cue, Pocahontas began singing the song, "Just Around the River Bend." I watched my kids go wide-eyed and semiconscious as the movie cast its spell. Relieved, I leaned back into the couch and turned my weary mind to the TV screen. And suddenly, before I knew it, I, the only adult in the room, was being whisked down the river in this vibrant flurry of song and animation as well.

And then it happened. Maybe because I was overtired, or maybe because I was an emotional basket case. But I associated so deeply with the final bars and scene of the song that I started to cry. Pocahontas had arrived at a fork in the river. The time was upon her to choose a path. Should she choose the river that appeared as smooth and steady as a beating drum? Or should she take a risk, go against her common sense, and choose the other, full of rapids and dreams and the unknown?

My heart pushed and pulled, as if being kneaded to the beat of the native drum. I felt every one of Pocahontas' words. I knew the position she was in. I'd arrived at a critical fork in *my* life's river, TWICE in the past two years: first, when Robert had an affair and I chose what I'd believed was the "smooth course," the safe route, by staying married. And then again, two years ago, when I chose the turbulent course, the one that broke all of society's rules and potentially put my reputation on the chopping block: I had an affair with Graham. And as I watched Pocahontas boldly take the more tumultuous river, even though everyone else had warned her not to, I felt her passion, her desire to reach for more, the fire in her heart and bones. And inwardly I applauded her. I applauded *myself*; not because I'm proud to have had an affair. But because I knew how much courage my choice had required. It went against everything I'd been taught or believed in. I'd had three kids and a family dream on board with me, and I was terrified. But I'd believed in love, I'd believed in me/us/destiny/the universe, and I'd dared to be true to my heart. And even though I didn't foresee the perilous waterfall of betrayal awaiting me ahead, even though I was *still* navigating an internal and external gulf of rapids, I wouldn't change any of my decisions.

I still had hope, *faith*, that somewhere up ahead, along this tumultuous, unbelted ride, I'd arrive at a place within myself that would make every second of this journey worthwhile; that somehow, in reaching new lows of sorrow, grief, failure, and fear, I'd one day be destined to reach heightened levels of joy and love; that each and every task, obstacle, and emotional danger I'd confronted along this course would change me, improve me, and empower me to live authentic to myself, not how the world expected me live.

"Are you crying Mom?" my five-year-old son suddenly asked, ducking his face in front of mine.

"Yeah," I replied, wiping my eyes with my sleeve.

"It's okay mom," he said sincerely, pulling my neck into a hug.

I chuckled, hugging him tenderly. "I'm not sad honey. It's just that . . . if you listen closely to the sound of the native drum, it opens up your heart."

And so I sat, snuggling with my children, to the very end of *Pocahontas*. And I cried many times throughout, as my heart throbbed to the not-so-steady rhythm of my own life. And when my children noticed my ongoing streams of tears, they nodded their heads sweetly . . . as if they understood.

CHAPTER 16

HOTEL FANTASY WITH A SERVICE MALE

Mission No. 5
Subject's Name: Patrick
Age: 28
Body Type: rugged and muscular
Penis Size: reported as 7 ½ inches long and 6 inches
around (unconfirmed)

WHEN PATRICK FIRST MESSAGED ME a month ago, his profile immediately seized my attention *and* made my imagination run wild. It read:

> Not looking for anything serious, just fun and intense. So tell me what you fantasize about, what you wish for and keep locked inside you. We'll keep it our secret . . .

Only one photo was attached: He was sitting on a curb in blue-jeans and a T-shirt, arm muscles were relaxed but bulging, his chiseled face and dark smoky eyes looked slightly off to the left. He was cloaked in an air of Mysterious Bad Boy. And I wanted to investigate.

Problem was, he lived and worked out of town. I doubted a face-to-face meeting would ever actually transpire. But then came his unexpected email: "I'm coming to town next Wednesday and staying at the Glenclose Hotel. Tell me what you want."

I saw fantasy written all over it: the backdrop, the circumstances, *and* the leading man. For over a decade, I'd secretly fantasized about lounging in a classy hotel bar, dressed to the nines, sipping white wine, and having a handsome, gallant man approach me. He'd buy me another drink and slowly engage me with his intelligence and charm (and killer smile). But I'd keep him guessing the whole time; the tango of seduction would be on.

But of course, he'd succeed, and we'd eventually end up in his hotel room for a long night of sensual, uninhibited pleasure. And the next day, after we kissed goodbye, I'd replay our delicious memories together. I knew I'd never see him again, and I'd be perfectly fine with that. Our one hot night together would fulfill my erotic fantasy.

Sure, I knew it seemed a little daring to want to live out this fantasy with an online stranger. The safer, more sensible choice would have been to role-play it within the safety of my marriage, or the cocoon of a love affair. After all, fantasies are supposedly best shared and explored with someone we trust and love, or so I was taught to believe.

The truth is, I never prioritized this fantasy when I was married or in love with Graham. More specifically, I didn't prioritize my Sexual Self, nor the process of getting to know that side of me more. Sure, I considered mentioning it to both of them, especially at the beginning of our relationships, when everything was new. But I couldn't summon my voice. I felt silly. Nervous, too. Beause what if they felt obliged rather than eager to enact it? What if the scene fell flat because they couldn't properly play their role, or it felt too contrived? I held this fantasy close to me, protectively, *self*-protectively; for in it, the man intuitively reads me. He gives me what I want, what I desire, what I yearn to feel . . . without instructions.

What further appealed to me was that the next day, I wouldn't have to do his laundry or listen to him belch in front of the TV.

While I knew I couldn't expect men to be mind-readers, and that I needed to verbalize my wants and preferences, I also believed a little focused intuition wasn't too much to ask for. Whether it was my husband or a stranger in a one-night fantasy, how hard could it be, I wondered, to bring more to the scene than a pant-load of testosterone? What about a little dash of imagination, a large heaping of confidence, mixed with a good dose of attention to nuance and subtlety? Because I knew I would intuit *his* every movement, gesture, smile, and word; I would *want* to make him feel like a Man. Call me entitled, but I didn't want to be skim-read like a box of cereal; making me feel like a Woman didn't just mean "wife" or "pussy." My feeling like a Woman should be his honor, his duty, and his ultimate pleasure.

But in order for anyone to "intuitively read" another person meant that his heart, on some level, must be open; mind/body energies needed to funnel through his heart center in order to access higher perceptions. And the men I'd been with to date didn't have a handle on that one. Most of their energy was concentrated solely between their legs. Maybe it's testosterone, maybe it's social conditioning about gender roles and expectations, or maybe they were so well taught to shove their emotions deep into their bellies (or into their muscles) that their heart passage remained underused, over guarded, or even out-of-order. Whatever the reason, I never got what I secretly yearned for, which, sadly, also robbed them from experiencing new levels of pleasure and intensity. Without intuition, the tango of seduction was reduced to the "Hokey Pokey."

Maybe I was aching for something that simply didn't exist. Maybe the steamy scenes I'd been fed through romance novels and erotic literature had mislead me, set unrealistic expectations about how men behaved, both romantically and sexually. I couldn't help but ask myself, if men *really* wanted to know what made women tick, why were they locked on hard-core porn sites instead of erotic literature. *Because men are visual,* my informed self told me. Yet, I just *knew* they were out there—men as sensual and playful and intuitive as me. I just had to find them.

But now, Patrick-with-the-smoky-eyes was not just coming to town, he was coming to a "hotel near me." It was time to realize my fantasy.

I wrote him an email outlining the seduction scene I wanted, deliberately saying nothing about sex. "You'll recognize me when you see me," I wrote. "But you must act like you don't know me. We are *complete strangers*. Your job will be to pick me up—and it won't be easy to win over a lady like me. You better be mentally ready to rise to the occasion and earn me . . . or you'll return to your hotel room alone."

He responded that he fully understood the scene and would perform his role expertly.

As I beautified for the evening and slipped on my lingerie and red wrap-dress, I inwardly groomed my starlet persona that I'd selected for my fantasy. She would shine in the lead role tonight and leave poor Patrick wondering, "Who *was* that incredible woman who shook my world?" Or at least that was my hope.

Driving to the hotel, I felt sexy, alive. This called for some Rihanna, a little "Good Girl Gone Bad." (Ha! It could be my new theme song!)

As I cranked the volume and sped down the highway, I sang along and meant every word of it. *I am SO the Good Girl Gone Bad,* I thought, laughing to myself. Wait, no-no-no-no-no. I'm worse! I am the Good *Stay-at-Home Mom* Gone Bad. Yup, that's right. We stay-at-home moms can get more than a little naughty too. But unlike our younger, child-free sisters, we are *extra* wise, *extra* strong, and we take whatever "extras" we want. You self-proclaimed "MILF" hunters have it all wrong—*we* aren't the prey, *you* are. You are but a *Service Male*—a SMILF!

And by the way, this SMILF huntress expects at least one orgasm before you have one.

. . . *And*, if I squirt and you have to change the sheets, I'll expect you to do so without complaint.

. . . And *and*—one last thing here since I'm on a roll: No. Small. Penises. Allowed.

WHILE PULLING INTO the hotel parking lot, I noticed a 7-11 in a strip mall close by. Pit stop: I needed cigarettes.

As I walked through the neon-lit store in my winter jacket, my strappy high heels clacking across the floor, heads turned in my direction. Inwardly I smiled: *That's a thumbs-up on the stunning factor, Houston!* Outwardly I beamed, my movements deliberate and unselfconscious.

Exiting the store, I noticed three men smoking and talking beside a parked car. I watched them literally halt their conversation midsentence to turn and stare at me.

Now in the past, such a reaction would have made me feel awkward and flustered. I'd have looked away as if I hadn't noticed them, or done something as idiotic as drop my car keys.

But not tonight. Instead, my vanity was empowering.

I stopped and faced them directly. "Hi guys, how are you?"

This time, *they* were the ones who became flustered and looked away embarrassed. "Good," one man managed to call out. They obviously weren't expecting the lady-object to speak.

I grinned and got back in my car. The alpha had emerged from the pack. And low and behold, it wasn't any of them, it was me. *Shane would be proud!* I felt suddenly so strong, independent, and in control. It was a pretty fabulous feeling.

Back in the hotel parking lot, I kept the engine running to

do a final mirror check: nose clear, no makeup smudges, fresh lipstick applied to moist lips. I was ready. I looked over at the hotel entranceway, wondering if Patrick was already inside.

Suddenly, the insanity of what I was doing hit me. *Have I lost my mind? Why am I doing this—and not Hali? Why am I the one who pushes things to the next degree? First there was Yummy Stranger, and now I'm planning to live out a fantasy with a total stranger?*

Who cares! I screamed to myself. *You're here now so get a move on. Walk the walk! Too many people talk the talk and never take action. Live it, do it, and analyze it tomorrow.*

I shut the car door and briskly walked into the hotel lobby. I easily followed signage to the bar and entered without pause.

I was greeted by the sound of classic rock music, the clink of cocktail glasses, and the hum of male conversation. Most of the stools were occupied—men in jeans and checkered work shirts or T's, who turned from their drinks to appraise me. *Damn, I'm way too overdressed for this place!* I thought panicked. I hadn't realized it was a popular hotel for oil rig workers.

But I straightened my shoulders and sidled up to the bar. *Screw it! Own your power,* I thought, as I ordered a glass of white wine. I deliberately kept my eyes facing front while the bartender poured. *I wonder if Patrick is watching me.* My spine tingled. *Play it cool*, I coached myself. *Remember, you're just some lovely diva who happened by this bar tonight. Act the role!*

Wine glass in hand, I strolled toward the back of the bar where it was quieter. He'd have to come find me over here; plan his approach, so-to-speak. While standing, I took my jacket off—slowly—imagining him watching me over a highball glass. *Damn, this is fun!* I thought, giddy with my newfound confidence. I couldn't believe I was actually finally doing this.

I sat poised and ladylike, casually drinking my white wine as if it was normal for a woman dressed like me to be in a place like this all alone. I could feel someone staring at me . . . I looked across a few tables and into the eyes of a bald-headed man with a big paunch. He looked like the archetype of a Mafia boss and so did his crew. *Give me a break,* I thought. His stare was so brazen, it was actually rude. He licked his upper lip. I stared right back, not smiling. *Who's gonna give?* I wondered. I felt feline and tough, sexy and powerful. *Tick-tock, tick-tock, tick-tock.* Finally, he half stood and waved. "Hi," he said, and then gave me a big dopey smile.

"Hi," I said back, with a nod of my head. I made no move to get up. He sat down and looked away. I sipped my wine. *Score another for Alpha Delaine!*

I fished through my purse to find my cell phone. Both Hali and Tory knew what I was up to. I had given them as many details as I could for my own protection. But I thought I should touch base with them, just to let them know all was well so far.

I'd almost finished dialing Hali's number when a man plopped down in the chair across from me. I looked up at him and thought, *Who are you?*

"Sorry I'm late!" the man before me said jovially. "I'm Patrick."

Slowly, I put down my glass and folded my arms in front of me. *What the . . . ?* This guy looked nothing like the guy online. He looked like a plump Islander from Hawaii, not a chiseled hunk.

Outwardly, I remained cool as my brain clamored to assess the situation. *I told him he was to pretend he didn't know me. And he came over and introduced himself as if this were a regular date. He broke my rule!*

"You don't look like your photo," I stated in a matter-of-fact tone.

"I don't?" He shifted in his seat.

I lifted my glass and took another sip. "No. You *don't.*" I continued to stare. He squirmed around some more, his round, soft cheeks smiling.

But his eyes were full of fear. I knew then, without a doubt, that this man could never mentally rise to my challenge.

After ten seconds of silence, he asked, "Do you want me to leave?"

Four-second pause.

"Yes."

And with that, he jumped off his chair and disappeared around the corner like he was doing the 100-meter dash.

I sat there stunned. My fantasy had gone directly from the starting gates to the finish line in under thirty seconds; a new world record, I'm sure.

Ten minutes later, I was driving home, *fuming,* a freshly lit cigarette scissored between my fingers. What a waste of time and energy! I'd been "had." He wasn't even who he said he was!

But despite my fuming, I suddenly giggled. The situation was just so *absurd.* And hilarious. Me in full fantasy mode, decked out, serious as could be about playing my "role"—and who cruises in but the antithesis of my "fantasy" hunk. Talk about crash and burn: that was fantasy *pulverization.*

Oh well, I thought with a grin. *Five gold stars to me for walking the talk. But I think it's time to reshelve this fantasy—too much of a wild card for the online dating world!*

And I swore I heard my guardian angels laugh, "Ya *think?*"

CHAPTER 17

A CHAMELEON IN SEARCH OF HOME

OVER THE PAST FEW WEEKS, both of my relationships with my service males—Adonis-Boy Daniel and Minotaur Brent—freefell to the ground at astonishing speeds. But there was no earth-shattering crash, no alarming 911 response. It was more like the sound of a shoulder shrug.

Perhaps if I'd maintained our relationships as dominant/submissive, as per Shane's instructions, the erotic mystique and "power" play may have lengthened their life spans. But when it came right down to it, I ended up just being me, which meant talking and getting to know them in a normal, friendly way outside the bedroom. As a result, our ten-year age difference flapped and crackled in my face like a wind-whipped red flag.

I tried to reserve judgment on them, to accept and appreciate them for exactly who they were. And I *did* see some good qualities in each of them, like Adonis Boy's flare for interior decorating, and Minotaur's fondness of cats. But our looking glasses were just too different; they'd never been married, neither had kids, and they were just getting started in their careers. In short, life was all about them.

"The key to making marriages work," Adonis Boy said to me on our third and final evening together, "is to not live together beforehand."

Great, I thought with a smile. *He's opening an interesting conversation.* "And . . . ?" I asked, waiting. "What else?"

"That's it," he said with a wave of his hand. "If you live together *before* the wedding, you've already bought pots and pans together and decorated your house. So after you sign the papers, nothing really changes. *But*, if you wait, you spend a good three years going out and shopping for pots and pans and stuff for your home. It's something new you can enjoy together."

Seriously?!

"But Daniel," I laughed, his naivety worse than I even imagined. "Down the road, life is going to throw you both many challenges— kids, work . . . and so many others. Whether you shopped for dishes before or after the wedding won't make a darn difference!"

"*No.* You're *wrong.*" Mouth pursed, he shook his blond head from side-to-side. "Couples just need to wait to move in together. It gives them the glue to stay together in the future."

Oh. My. God. He *was* serious. I had to turn my face away as he then *pontificated* to me about marriage and divorce. His ignorance and righteousness were too much—with each slow blink of my eyes, his golden Adonis aura was fading.

A few days later, I saw Minotaur Brent for the third and final time, too. He'd had a long, stressful day at work. I knew he was grumpy (he was a moody type), so I let him spew for a while as we sat on the couch. Then, true to Delaine form, I offered up words of support and empathy: "I know what you're saying, Brent. My stress level often goes into the red zone, too. But it'll pass. Try to let it go till tomorrow."

He laughed, "What stress do *you* know? You're just a stay-at-home mom."

Raw nerve exposed. My eyes shifted from side-to-side. *Relax, Delaine. He's not Robert. He's just young and ignorant. He doesn't mean anything by it.*

"You have no idea . . . " I said to the wall, willing myself not to lay into him.

But fifteen minutes later, I still hadn't recovered. He was no longer a Minotaur but an arrogant, ignorant donkey's ass. Suffice to say, I didn't see him again.

What killed me now, in retrospect, was how poorly I'd reacted to their egotism. Inwardly, I was appalled and screaming, but outwardly, I avoided conflict. Moreover, I saw how, in a few other conversations we shared, I not only "dumbed myself down" to appeal to their level, but I also brushed off insensitive comments to "keep the peace."

So much for Dominant Tough Girl.

Why couldn't I muster my alpha side? I knew she was there. Was the chameleon-like Delaine who sat across from these boys more concerned with winning their approval than being true to her convictions and who she was? Or had my marriage trained me to brush off rudeness, chauvinism, even callousness to avoid conflict and disharmony? Maybe I was simply hardwired to want to please others at the expense of my authentic self. But I had to wonder, who the heck *was* the authentic Delaine anyway? I knew she was in there somewhere. Perhaps the first step to becoming more real was becoming aware of when I *wasn't*.

I always thought my "chameleon" inclination was a good thing—that it made me adaptable, more expansive, and better able to connect and *blend* with different types of people. But upon closer examination, I also recognized its shadow side: the loss of my own true colors. I'd been wearing camouflage for so long, I couldn't even remember what the vibrant shades of myself looked like. Because this chameleon-like tendency undermined my true self when I dealt with domineering personalities. Like Robert. I became compliant and acquiescent. In fact, with Robert, I'd have bent myself into a pretzel if it meant keeping him happy or keeping the peace.

Oh, you need to stay out all night and get drunk with your friends? Sure, Robert darling, go ahead. I'll drive home alone and pay the baby sitter. I'll get up in the middle of the night with the kids.

What's that? You'll need to sleep it off in the morning? Of course, honey, I'll bring the kids out somewhere first thing so the house will be quiet. 'K, have a good time, sweetheart.

How often had that scenario played itself out? Once, twice a month? Or had it *really* been every other night when he was home, just in more subtle ways? God, why hadn't I just said, "Nope, you get your butt home. You should be with your wife and kids!" But I hadn't. I'd just bent. Despite the cost to me.

When it came to arguing with Robert, my vertebrae were as supple as unbaked dough. It wouldn't matter what we were at odds about, the dynamic was almost always the same: I would carefully approach him, and clearly, but sincerely, express my concerns— I didn't want to come across as on the attack. But his response was almost always the same: passive-aggressive anger. He'd go into internal lockdown, ignoring me, avoiding me, throwing back-handed remarks at me. Potent one-liners, full of disdain. I hated it. I hated the tension; I hated the knot in my stomach; I hated the fact that we were wasting the precious limited time we had together in between his work assignments.

So *I* would apologize to *him*. Apologize for bringing it up, apologize for making him mad or upset. *Yes, honey, I know you work hard when you're out of town . . . Yes I know you're a great provider and you're doing the best you can . . . Yes, I'm just being silly. Yeah, stubborn and unreasonable, too. What's that? Make up sex? Yeah . . . sure . . .*

I definitely needed to get a handle on my knee-jerk deference response, not just with the men I dated, but with Robert. Because he was *still* threatening and bullying me around our separation agreement. A part of me wanted to cave in to his financial terms just so I could free myself from him and move on with my life.

Yet another part of me screamed, *Stand your ground, Delaine! He is so accustomed to you giving in to him that he assumes he'll get his way again. You need this money to look after yourself and your kids, and whether he likes it or not, he has a financial responsibility to you.*

So I wasn't going to cave. I still *wavered* from time to time, but I wasn't backing down.

Lately, when I'd had contact with Robert, I did a little creative visualization to help me deal with him: I'd metamorphose into my Warrior Woman, a respected and close ally of my Wild Woman. I'd imagine myself standing before him in a warrior stance with a shield in my hands, instead of my hands wrapped defensively around my chest. I'd look him square in the eyes and hold his gaze, instead of looking away. Still, sometimes I exited our meetings wounded all the same, and it took me a few days to recover. But sometimes not. And I walked away with my head held high.

As I employed this tactic, I noticed changes in his behavior. He avoided looking me in the eyes more. Hey, for all I know, maybe the sight of me disgusted him. But my intuition said he sensed I was getting stronger. I sensed his growing cowardice. And yet . . . my softer, more forgiving side was a strong force too, because while I felt proud of the progress I was showing, I nonetheless felt compassion and sympathy for him; he, too, was struggling to figure out life as a newly single father. But I knew I couldn't let my guard down about the settlement and custody agreements. He'd come in for the jugular every time.

As for my brief "relationships" with Adonis Boy Daniel and Minotaur Brent, I had no regrets. Unwittingly, they helped me take a deeper look at my chameleon-like nature. And they enticed me to step out of the "Land of Shouldn'ts" and into harmless Young Man Territory. Their sexually desiring me was a great ego rub; no doubt about that. And having sex with them was good, delicious fun. Not only did I expend my pent-up sexual energy on them, but I also discovered I could G-spot orgasm in different positions and with different men other than with Football Coach Chad and his "maneuver." It ultimately affirmed that *I was* the one in charge of my body; my body, my sexuality, and my sensuality belonged to me.

My young-man relationships also confirmed something that I already knew: A nice butt and a broad set of shoulders weren't enough to hold my interest for long. I could respect and appreciate them for all their worth to me, but I was definitely ready to move on.

The question was . . . to what?

THE "THOUGHT" CROSSED my mind today. It wasn't the first time. In fact, it had stuck its nose in my face hundreds of times since I'd initiated my divorce.

Maybe I should get back together with Robert.

Doubts always lurked around my decision to end my marriage: *What if I gave up too soon? What if things got better? What if, what if, what if?*

Sometimes I wished I hated him; then all doubt would be eradicated. If I could dump all my anger, blame, and hurt on top of him, I could turn him into a monster so hideous that I could wallow, self-righteously, in the role of Undeserving Victim. But I knew it didn't work that way, that hate would only turn its ugly head on me and eat me from the inside out. My wish was nothing but an illusion, a fantasy of a quick fix that momentarily justified my suffering and excused me from having to take responsibility. For anything.

But I knew I still loved Robert in many ways, in spite of how unkind he could be. It was my nature to see the best of a person, to their core. And I believed in his authentic goodness. I would always care about him. I simply didn't have enough rage to wipe out all our wonderful memories together. I couldn't label him Evil when I could still feel the warmth of his smiles and laughter. Or when I remembered the times he cried, the times he tenderly held my children, the times he generously gave with his love and money. I couldn't take the vastness of his spirit and lock it into a container marked "POISON."

Thoughts are funny things—dangerous too. My conscious mind never seems to turn off. It's an endless barrage of memories, analyses, projections, fantasies. It chatters to the point of overload, determined to understand, decipher, solve. And quick on its heels lay an army of emotions, a chaotic mass of furious feelings that range from love and gratitude to anger and despair. I become prisoner to an internal hell that is 100 percent self-created. Could Robert and I salvage our marriage? Could we have a decent life together if we chose to? I knew the answers were yes. It would take a tremendous amount of work, but yes, we could. But the bigger, more important question remained: Was Robert the man I wanted, desired, and deserved to spend my life with?

I loved Robert when I married him. My definition of love back then was more naïve and more limited than what it is now, but my feelings for him were genuine. Often I hear divorced people speak bitterly about their marriage: that it was a mistake, that they never really loved their ex, that warning signs had been flashing from the get-go. My hindsight exposed those incongruities, too. But I felt no need to minimize or rip apart a love I deemed so beautiful in my twenties. It was real to me then and offered me many gifts, like my three beautiful children. If a marriage was already dead, why wave a carving knife over its grave?

I found myself constantly pondering the meaning of "true love." Through TV, books, my family, the church, I was indoctrinated to believe it was the ultimate goal in life, that it was this magical merging of two souls on every level. And that "time" was one of its essential ingredients—a lifetime, that is. No doubt, there was something beautifully romantic and courageous in the idea of two people witnessing each other's entire life journey, through all the triumphs and heartbreaks.

But I wasn't convinced that that definition was correct. And I felt certain I was but one of thousands, if not millions, who had questioned it. Especially if they'd gone through a divorce. I wondered if perhaps true love wasn't something conferred on you by another, but that it was more a state of personal being that one expressed outwardly and received in return. A state of being that was not exclusive, but *inclusive*: to her partner, her friends, her neighbors, her coworkers, and the vast beautiful world at large. To me, *that* kind of love seemed the ultimate, for it honored the connectedness and sacredness of all life.

My personal take on this thing called life is that we're here on Earth to learn and grow and evolve into beings of love— individually. Perhaps that process is fostered within one serious relationship alone, or not. If a relationship no longer served me on a spiritual level, I wondered, should I feel compelled, guilty, obliged to stay in it—whether I made those vows two, five, or twenty years ago? Do the rules and expectations of marriage sabotage our souls' ultimate mission?

I couldn't help but wonder if this reluctance to let go of a relationship when it became detrimental rather than nourishing was because of our perception of death. Whether it's the death of relationship or the death of anything else, I always perceived it as an awful thing I had to resist, fight, or oppress. But death is intrinsic to life. Maybe I'd clung to the idea of marriage not just out of love, but out of fear. By vowing to stay together "till death do us part," I believe I felt a little less vulnerable in the face of the unknowable future. Safety in numbers, comfort in my husband *and* our children.

But my feelings evolved. I now understood that death was a period of transformation, not annihilation. That within the ashes of death lay the seeds of new growth, new learning, new opportunities for the self. I no longer could reduce it to black and white—that life was "good" and death was "bad."

And I needed to apply this insight now.

So I asked myself again: What do I really want? Not what my fear said I should want, or what society said I should want, but what this soul named Delaine wanted. On one side of the tee-ter-totter sat a single mother of three, facing an unknown future all alone. *She was terrified!* Across from her sat an emotionally exhausted mom/wife fighting to save a dying marriage riddled with wounds.

I tried to imagine what it would be like to sit across from Robert again as his wife. And all I saw was a man heavily chained, a prisoner of his upbringing, his closed-down emotions, his take on what it meant to be a man. I saw myself looking at him, trying to break down his walls, knowing that within that steely shell lay an abundant, feeling, beautiful soul. I *knew* that it was there: I'd caught glimmers of it in his eyes, and sometimes it spread to his voice and his actions and we connected in a higher way.

But inevitably, without cause or word of warning, his walls would seal back up. He was gone. Once again, I found myself powerless—my hopes, needs, dreams were sucked into that chasm, too. I wanted to grab him by the shoulders and scream: *Open up your soul for God's sake! Can't you see that's the most beautiful part of who you are!* But I didn't. Instead, I turned my pain and frustration within . . . and then I'd turned to Graham. How could I back step so far and find happiness? I couldn't. I would simply blend again in his presence.

My mind overloaded, I exhaled away my thoughts and brought my awareness inside my body. There was just one more question to ask, the one I ultimately returned to navigate my course of action: *Could I ever enjoy sex again with Robert?*

The answer was fast and visceral: my stomach clenched, my body tensed, and my inner thighs moved to close. The answer was an indisputable "*No.*"

And so I threw my hands up in surrender. My head and heart just couldn't figure things out. I had to trust that my body knew things that the rest of me still didn't.

CHAPTER 18

THEY JUST WEREN'T THAT INTO US

I FINALLY MADE A DECISION about what I *really* wanted in a relationship right now: a "friend with benefits." I knew I wasn't ready for the demands of a fully committed love relationship—I was still getting over old pains, after all—but I did want ongoing sex with *one* open-minded, decent man. Yes, one.

Football Coach Chad was someone I could have seen in this role: we laughed a lot, we grew up in the same *era*, and, topping it off like hot chocolate sauce, he was a deliciously fine lover.

The problem was, he hadn't called. In over *five weeks*. This time I wasn't making any excuses for him. Even if he called me tomorrow, there was no way I'd see him again. I didn't want an arrangement that happened but once a month and on someone else's terms.

My only consolation was knowing that Hali was as confused about the concept as I was. A couple of weekends ago, she'd met a prime candidate for the position: Payton, the wavy-haired computer techie I'd left squirming in the parking lot. Yup, I'd played matchmaker *again*.

When Hali had first spoken with Payton by phone, she'd been in one of *those* moods: ravenous for sex and too impatient to pretend otherwise. "*No*, I don't want to go out to a movie," she'd said, when he suggested one. "*No*, I don't want you to rent a movie either. I want you to come to my house tonight so we can see what our chemistry is like. I only have one thing on my mind." Payton had been startled by her directness but had eagerly played along.

But boundaries got skewed when their initial night of partying between the sheets turned into a weekend-long bacchanal of sex, friendship, *and* romance. They spent every waking and sleeping minute together, shopping, cooking, and even running errands.

But ten days had now passed, and he hadn't phoned or tried to see her again. He had avoided her online and only sometimes responded to her text messages.

"I just don't get it," Hali said angrily. We were commiserating over the phone while I watched my kids through the window as they played on my front lawn. I sipped my cup of tea as she spoke. "I know I was bold with him the first night. But we spent the whole weekend together—he saw other sides of me, the *real* me, and he really liked me! I even apologized for being so direct with him that first night and explained that I don't normally act that way. He'd said it turned him on to have a woman assert herself like that."

Together, Hali and I wracked our brains trying to figure out our situations: hers with Computer-Techie Payton, mine with Football Coach Chad. We dug deeper: *What weren't we understanding?* We wondered aloud if the old-school rules still strongly applied when it came to dating and sex. Should we wait for a man to call us after our first liaison, even if all we wanted was sex and a little company? Maybe this friends with benefits concept was a myth or, at best, a rarity? We were discouraged, to say the least.

"Maybe guys just can't handle it when they know a woman primarily wants sex from them," Hali offered. "I think they like the idea superficially, but it ends up challenging their masculinity, you know?"

"Yeah," I agreed. "But I also wonder if you and I intimidate men, Hali. I mean, we're not only attractive, intelligent, and classy—excuse me, but we *are*—" I added, chuckling, "we're also confident enough to express our needs and call the shots sexually. I'm not sure guys know what to do with us or make of us. Maybe they'd be more comfortable if we were as naïve and needy as we were when we were younger."

"Maybe," said Hali. "That, or they think we're slutty or desperate. It would be easier for them to fall back on judging us instead of facing their own glaring insecurities."

I sighed. "You know, I really thought the rules had changed and women were so much more empowered these days," I said. "But I think the old double standard is still in effect."

"Totally," Hali agreed.

I paused for a moment. "Maybe deep down men simply need to be the 'hunters,'" I continued. "And when they become the hunted, their manhood is rattled. All I know for sure is that at my age, I think I should be entitled to express my sexual wants. And instead, I'm sitting here feeling like a teenager, wondering, 'What is he thinking? Why hasn't he called?' It makes me think there's something wrong with me and I really resent that."

"It's rejection, right?" she said. "And rejection sucks no matter what. But we can't take it out on ourselves. I chose to be daring with Payton because that's what I wanted, and it felt right at the time. Maybe another man would have reacted differently. Whatever." Hali paused. "The bottom line is that we don't know where these guys are coming from, so we shouldn't take it personally." She was right.

Suddenly my call waiting bleeped. I looked at the number, "Hali, Tory's on the other line. She's trying to book tickets for a show in Vegas next week so I better go."

"Man, I sure wish I was going with you all," Hali said longingly. Then: "*Pfft*—at least in Vegas you'll know exactly what the rules are: There are none!"

I smiled as I clicked through to Tory. *I was counting on it.*

THE NEXT DAY Hali phoned me again, this time much more upbeat. "I picked up a book at Chapters last night called *He's Just Not That into You.* It gives all sorts of clues into the male psyche. Listen to this:

"Wake-up call Number 41: 'Men don't forget how much they like you. So put down the phone.'"

Hali laughed. I heard her flipping pages through the book. She continued: "Number 59: 'If he's not calling you, it's because you are not on his mind.'"

Hmmmm, I thought to myself. *It makes sense. But is it really that simple?*

As if hearing my question, Hali then read: "'Number 10: Men are not complicated, although we'd like you to think we are.' That's true, eh? They really *are* simple creatures. We're *way* deeper and more complex than them. Smarter, too," she laughed.

"Hold on, here's another one: 'If the guy you're dating doesn't seem to be completely into you, or you feel the need to start 'figuring him out,' please consider the glorious thought that he might just not be that into you. And then free yourself to go find someone that *is*.'"

I listened attentively. Though amusing, these points were very poignant.

"Oh, and I love this one, Delaine. 'Number 116: Cheaters are people who have a lot of stuff to work out, and they're working it out on *your* time and with *your* heart.' Man, that's so true, isn't it?"

"Absolutely," I replied wryly, thinking of both Graham and Robert. Suddenly, I looked at the time: "Hali, I have to bring the kids to swimming lessons. I'll call you back tonight."

A half-hour later, I sat among parents in the swimming pool bleachers, thinking about the insights from Hali's book. Essentially, they clearly spelled out what I already knew: When a man is interested in you, not even a herd of elephants will stop him from pursuing you. I know this is true because I'm the same way when

I'm into someone. *Time to stop making excuses for any man; and call it for what it is,* I thought. "That he's just not into me."

When I looked back on my history with men, including before marriage, one thing was blatantly clear: I'd wasted a hell of a lot of time and energy trying to figure men out: What were they thinking? How could I help them, understand them, fix them? It had been my personal quest to make them healthy, whole, and happy. Heck, when I was married, I'd made Robert's happiness my *responsibility.* Somewhere along the way, I'd decided that my wife job included not only being his best friend, but also his twenty-four-hour therapist, his spiritual counselor, and of course, his perpetually available pussy. Soul, mind, body—whatever his needs were—even the ones he wasn't aware of, my job was to be the supreme caretaker.

And all the while, my fingers were anxiously crossed behind my back, hoping, wishing, *begging* for him to see what a wonderful woman I was. I was a disaster waiting to happen; a doormat being weaved. Because as soon as Robert—or any other man I dated—brushed me off or disrespected me, guess what I did? I immediately blamed myself, of course, as if somehow *I* was the one lacking something: compassion, intuition, guts, desirability, sexiness, spiritual insight . . . I took it personally, straight to the heart, as if I was at fault for not measuring up. Never did it cross my mind that maybe we just didn't fit, that the problem was theirs alone, that I was amazing as I was, or that maybe, just maybe, I damn well deserved *better.*

But I was finally realizing that now. I also realized that now was the perfect time for me to stop being such a shape shifter and be more solid in who I was. Any man who dated me was one heck of a lucky guy, and if he couldn't be bothered to woo me, respect me, and for God's sake, *call* me when he said he would, then he could take the express route to Jerk-Off Land. I'd settled for less for way too long. That road would end here.

CHAPTER 19

ADVENTURES IN WONDERLAND

APPARENTLY, SHANE ENROLLED ANOTHER "student'" in his online alpha-training classroom: a twenty-seven year old master's student at UCLA named Lynn. According to Shane, not only was she a "much better listener" than me, her success outside the classroom had earned her major gold stars: Not only did she have one guy scrubbing her toilet and doing her laundry, she'd manipulated some rich trust-fund boy into paying her to be his "faux-girlfriend" at public events.

I admit I was somewhat fascinated with my classmate's arrangements—in a *wow, I can't-believe-people-actually-did-that* kind of way. But they simply didn't jive with me: my morals, my principles, or my stay-at-home mom lifestyle. My home—my *kids'* home—would never be that kind of playground. Thus, I sent him an email to put my foot down and close the conversation:

> Listen, I'm NOT going to continue arguing with you about whether it's right or wrong to "devour" dik-dik men. The bottom line is that that's not how I see submissive men. To me, they're more like yipitty lapdogs that I'd prefer to have go away. I don't need anyone to wash

my car or hang around begging for ways to service me. So let's simply agree to disagree.

I've decided I'm going to try and find a "friends with benefits" relationship to satisfy my sexual appetite. At the same time, I'm keeping my eyes open for a dominant alpha male—a man more my equal who could hold my interest. (I know of one in New York, but he won't even send me a photo.) Who knows . . . maybe I could even dominate HIM.

The countdown to my Vegas trip is on! Me and the girls are leaving in three days. It'll be my first time there. Wonder if I'll get up to any mischief . . .

His reply arrived just before I signed off for bed.

Delaine:

I will expect a full slut report when you get back from Vegas.

Once you're home we can discuss your coming here, assuming you are still wet . . .

Underneath Shane's email was a photo of him, from the waist up. *Hmmm.* I sat back in my chair and stared at his picture: "*Finally,*" I said aloud. "Hello there, Shane."

He certainly didn't look like anyone I'd pick out in a bar. He'd lost most of his grayish-brown hair (Dr. Phil-style), he had a trimmed moustache, and he even had a belly. But somehow that neither surprised nor bothered me.

I leaned forward in my chair and stared into the dark eyes looking out from the screen. "Who *are* you?" I whispered aloud. I examined his eyes closely, looking for clues, insights into the man behind them. I closed my eyes for a moment, imagining his hefty, six-foot-three frame towering over me. I felt him grab me by the back of my hair and how I would look up at him (my eyes flew open) into *those* dark eyes.

Excitement rippled through my body. What wicked things might he have me do? What power would he unleash over me and unto me? The answers lay hidden behind those eyes. I could feel his dominance, the intensity of his size and energy, his voice in my ear as his hands claimed me as his own. I would submit to his every wish and desire.

Yes. I sat up tall in my chair. There was no doubt in my mind. I *was* attracted to this man.

Then: *Holy shit. He wants me to go meet him in New York!*

WHAT A SIGHT we were: seven sexy, late-thirty-something women going to Sin City. United States' Customs was a ghost town as we passed through it, strutting, laughing, pulling our carryons side by side and row by row. We were so abuzz with excitement, we were like a tiny swarm of honeybees as we made our way to the already packed gate. And like every other person destined for Las Vegas, we'd paid special attention to how we looked—as if the moment we stepped off the plane, we'd step immediately into party central. I couldn't believe I had once thought our age bracket was old; we made it look so good! I looked around at the glowing faces of my girlfriends and I knew, I just *knew*, this would be an unforgettable trip. Because we weren't just fresh-faced innocents with few responsibilities walking that tarmac to an adult playground, we were women with families, careers, love and loss, and even wisdom. We were responsible. Abandon didn't come easy, but that's what we were hoping to do for this small pocket of days. *Live with abandon.*

So who were we? Tory, my former roommate was here, as well as Patty, my stunning, "older" girlfriend who had kindly "connected me" with Yummy Stranger during my time of "need." Also joining us was our close friend Selena, a married mom who some-how always breathed of style and sophistication, even when her kids were first born and she was covered in spit up. And a handful of others who were just as dear and important to me. We'd come to know each other over a decade ago through dinners and birthday celebrations (ours, not our kids), and somehow, almost magically, strong and special friendships had formed, both individually, and collectively. We'd seen each other through major milestones: some of us had become mothers, some had excelled along career paths, a few had seen a marriage or relationship come apart. We'd drifted apart periodically, sometimes for a year at a time, but somehow we'd always returned to one another, to our group, where there was a sense of freedom and love that was as grand and unique as our summed personalities.

Prior to leaving on our trip, Tory had expressed that she was a little nervous about all of us vacationing together. After all, we'd never done this before—nowadays, longer trips had only trans-pired with husbands, partners, and/or kids. What if we got on each other's nerves? What if, because we were older, we'd become more anal and less tolerant in ways we didn't realize? Would our personalities clash when we were mashed together in the same hotel room? My mind flashed to girl vacations from my early twenties; there had definitely been times of friction. But surely, we had grown up.

By eleven o'clock the night we arrived, we'd finished beautify-ing en masse in our suites and were ready to hit the town. First up on the agenda was a club called Pure, where tables were reputed to cost upward of eight-hundred dollars a night. Tory, the minx, had scored us free entrance tickets. And as we stood in line at the VIP entrance, gambling machines bleeping and singing around us, I took in the vibrant action around me. It *was* like landing on another planet. Half-dressed showgirls with epic breasts and glittery attire sauntered through the casino halls, grabbing everyone's attention, including my own. I couldn't help but feel a little plain in comparison. But I was happy with how I looked: my brown and gold dress hung elegantly just past my knees and showed off my slim figure and tear-drop bustline. My hair was down and full of soft, loose curls. I felt sexy, but classy, which aligned with the kind of man I hoped to meet that night: a handsome, successful, refined *man*—no boys allowed on this trip!

Pure was packed, wall to wall, back to front. As we inched our way through the downstairs bar, bodies bumped and grinded and rubbed, both on the dance floor and off. Alcohol was flowing, flesh was bare for an eyeful, and a mood of "anything goes" infused the air.

I stood to the side of the bar, trying not to grimace as I sipped my white wine (at eighteen dollars a glass, it was going down, like it or not) and took in the room in an out-of-body way. I felt like Alice in Wonderland; like I'd just fallen into an adult playground in some parallel universe. Sure, millions of people visit Vegas every year—I was no different—but it felt no less exotic and surreal to me than if I really was the first suburban stay-at-home mother to ever land here. I couldn't believe it was Sunday night. A *Sunday!* Bath night for the kids, Sunday dinner, getting lunches and backpacks ready for a new week of school, slip into my Super Girl jammies, and hit the hay. If this was Vegas on a Sunday night, *whoa.* What would Friday look like? *The world didn't suddenly stop having fun, Delaine, just because you chose to stay home and have babies,* a voice teased inside my head. I could definitely see how one's sense of time and morality could quickly disappear in a place like this—hedonism was not governed by a clock!

Half an hour later, my girlfriends had scattered into the crowd and I was standing by myself, feeling removed. The crowd seemed so young, the men like university students. I hungered for a classier experience. And frankly, there were no chairs and my feet were pissed off to be in heels instead of comfy mom flats.

Suddenly, my girlfriend Shannon appeared beside me. "Delaine," she said, excitedly, grabbing my free hand. "You need to come with me; I can get us into a private party on the patio upstairs!" I eagerly followed her up three flights of stairs, past two huge bouncers, and through red-cordoned rope. If anyone could maneuver her way into a private VIP function it would be her. Shannon, whom I'd become fast friends with when we first met twelve years ago at a fitness club where we both taught aerobics, always stood out wherever she went. Tall and blonde, with a smile that could turn dictators into diplomats, she attracted men and attention like a magnet. With her added attributes of height, style, and a voluptuous figure, not to mention a kind, engaging personality, she could charm anyone, including Pure's 250-pound bouncers.

Now *this* was where I wanted to be. Partying on the other side of the velvet ropes meant elbowroom, comfy black leather couches, and free decanters of wine and highballs that were never left empty. Soon we were being courted—not by young drunk boys, but by a crowd of sharp-dressed men over thirty-five. They quickly informed us they were part of an exclusive entrepreneurial association for millionaires. *That explains the pricey suits and tuxes,* I thought. But were they telling us the truth? *Pfft. Who cares!* I liked their story, so I bought it with a container of salt.

I slid onto a couch overlooking the roof, the bright lights of Vegas sparkling around me in the warm night air. A man across from me quickly refilled my wine glass. As I thanked him, a dark-haired stranger wearing an elegant suit and pink silk tie sat down on the cushion beside me. He reached out his large, manicured hand and smiled warmly. "Good evening," he said. "Please allow me to introduce myself. My name is Anton." I met his dark eyes, and I felt instant attraction. I thought, *Helloooooo, Anton!*

The next few hours were a blur. I spent most of it sitting and talking to Anton, with frequent bathroom breaks to sneak smokes and consume copious amounts of Tic Tacs. Shannon had smuggled the rest of the girls across the red line and they, too, quickly lost themselves in the free-flowing alcohol and predominantly male VIP gathering.

By night's end (maybe 4:00 AM?), a few of us girls were still up on the rooftop, but we had migrated into what appeared to be a Mongolian tent. Inside its privacy, on a u-shaped couch full of cushions, I watched, smiling, as my friends talked and flirted with a handful of new male friends. Faces aglow, we were at our sultry best—relishing not just our femininity, but the sweet novelty of the moment; I wanted to capture it in a snow globe and keep it on a shelf. Beside me, Anton had loosened his pink silk tie (damn that was one nice tie!) and relaxed into the couch with his legs stretched out and crossed. Through my drunken lens, he looked like an Arabian prince. I was more than aware of his arm around me and our legs touching. I caught Tory's eye and she gave me a look that said, *Girl, you'd be a fool not to take advantage of that luscious man beside you.* I looked at Anton, and his dark eyes held me, filled with seductive calm and intention. I had no doubt that his full Mediterranean lips and strong hands would consume me entirely. This was no service boy. I didn't need any of Tory's encouraging. I'd already made up my mind . . .

A limo ride back to his hotel, the push and pull of stops and corners, as his full lips pressed on mine the entire way there. Experienced, hungry, sensual. My memories of that night are like snapshots spilled across a table: A lavish hotel suite, the biggest I've ever been in. Him draping his pink silk tie over the back of a chair. Him walking towards me, white shirt unbuttoned and flowing, like a God walking the shores of the sea. Strong arms lifting me onto the dresser and my body flowering under his hands and wet lips.

Being lifted again . . . and carried to the bed. The sound of a package opening (protection!). His warm gaze on my face as he took me in his arms yet again.

My memory of the sex we shared is limited to the missionary position: his powerful back flexing on top of me, his moans in my ear, my mounting pleasure. I remember having an orgasm, and that it was delicious and lusty, but I don't remember how long the sex lasted or if *he* even had an orgasm.

Truth be told, I pretty much passed out.

Yeah. Totally and completely.

But soon after, I woke up wondering where I was. I looked over at Anton, still fast asleep beside me. *Still unbelievably handsome!* Dim snippets from the night began replaying in my brain. And I still felt drunk; my head was fuzzier than my son's favorite lovey.

Daylight was just starting to stream in through the French doors. *Look at that view of the city!* I thought, enchanted. Then: *Hmmm, I wonder what happened to all my girlfriends . . .*

Quietly, s-l-o-w-l-y, so as not to wake him, I slid out of bed, picked up my strewn clothes, and redressed. At first I worried about walking out in the bright early morning in a sultry evening dress, and then I remembered it was Vegas! I'd blend right in . . .

I'm not sure what compelled me, but I'd decided to leave without a trace. I'd slip out of his bedroom, out into the massive crowds of Vegas, and disappear from his life. I knew it was both nervy and rude. But it felt right. And exciting. We'd had our night of passion, and that's what we were after. Nothing more. It had been glitzy, romantic, and incredibly racy and fun. But *I* wanted to decide how this story would end; it was like an updated version of my Hotel Fantasy. I knew we'd never be ongoing lovers. Simply "disappearing" seemed the perfect ending to a magical night.

So I softly closed the door behind me. And vanished.

LIKE ANY GROUP of women that "experiences" Vegas with gusto, we girls flew home with our own stories of silliness and drunken mischief. Like when we deliberately cat-walked down the casino's red carpets using Hali's famous "grocery store stripper walk." Or when a few of us drank vodka with Red Bull for the first time and laid claim to any piece of open carpet as our dance floor. Or when we crammed three of us at a time into the changing room of Frederick's of Hollywood, trying on rhinestone-covered lingerie.

But in my eyes—and heart, as I looked around at my girl-friends on our plane ride home—I knew we'd experienced something "extra" special, even *profound* on our trip. And I wasn't alone in that "feeling": Tory said she felt "changed," Selena said she felt her husband "was going to sense I'm different and I won't know how to explain it." And Patty said she felt more "powerful . . . grounded," attributing it entirely to our group's energy. But even if we couldn't put our fingers exactly on it, it was real and it was powerful. I felt beautiful, I felt alive, and felt like I was not just a part of a whole but more whole. In allowing myself to rise up and free my Fabulous Self, I'd become fabulously free.

BUT THAT FREE-SPIRITED high didn't last long. Within seventy-two hours of being home from Vegas, I emotionally crashed. I wasn't a total wreck, but my "Fabulous Self" had to squeeze back into the contained bottle of "Same-old Daily Self."

What further zapped the winds from my sails was my next phone conversation with Shane. We'd started out on the right track, sharing laughs over my Vegas stories, including my drunken encounter with Anton. But then, as our conversation switched to me flying to New York and I expressed my intention of bringing my own hotel money "just in case," he became rather quiet. I sensed he was even . . . annoyed?

"Delaine, you do know why you're coming here, right?" he asked softly.

"Yes," I replied. "First and foremost to spend time with you. I'm really looking forward to talking to you and picking that crazy mind of yours!"

Silence on the other end. He was waiting.

"And *maybe* we'll have sex," I added, with a nervous laugh.

"Delaine, you *do* understand that I am a Dominant, and you'll be here to submit to me."

"Yes, Shane. I know you're the 'Super Alpha Male.' But I also know you aren't into freaky stuff and you won't hurt me. *If* it even comes down to us having sex."

"No, I would never hurt you. But you need to understand that certain things will be required of you should we connect. For example, on your third night here, if we haven't already, I will want anal sex."

Now, I'm no prissy, and I've nothing against folks who enjoy anal sex, but during our months of correspondence, Shane had openly shared his penis size with me. And it was *very* large. He claimed it was nine inches long and six inches in circumference. At the time I was thrilled: He'd be Super Alphalicious to crawl on top of.

But anal sex? *Are you kidding me?!* The thought downright scared me.

"Anal sex is important to me," he continued. "I need to know you can take it. Not 'kind of' take it, with a grimace on your face or you needing me to stop because it hurts. But take it like a *real* woman."

Long pause, even a bristle. I knew he was baiting me.

"I just can't give you that kind of guarantee, Shane. I can't even guarantee we'll have *regular* sex. I'm not experienced with anal sex and I don't even know if I'll like it. I really don't know how I feel about the whole thing. But I definitely have my doubts."

Our conversation thus came to an abrupt and unexpected halt.

I hung up the phone in shock. This phone call was to have finalized our plans, not throw a monkey wrench into them.

I shook my head in disbelief. After all these months of talking and emailing, we had ended it because of a stalemate over anal sex?

I awoke the next morning feeling deflated. I checked my inbox, hoping he had written. But of course, he hadn't. The bottom line was that he had clear expectations around what he wanted, and I had equally clear boundaries of my own. Our meeting was off.

I was surprised by how our disagreement affected me. I'd grown attached to Shane these past months, and while I knew we lived three thousand miles apart, I felt his presence in my life almost daily: his raw sexual power, his mentoring and friendship, his shocking sense of humor. I knew I'd miss him.

Even though our "relationship" was a little on the bizarre side, there was no denying I'd grown tremendously from it. He exposed me to a new way of perceiving and thinking, of viewing sexuality and the world at large. I learned to take risks, to step into my sexuality, and assert myself more in mind and body. I learned to stop apologizing for breathing, and to stop caring so much about what everyone else thought. In essence, he helped me give *myself* permission to explore new aspects of who I was. Without him, I doubt that would have happened, at least not as quickly or to such a degree. In fact, had he not been *exactly* who he was—an intelligent, zany, sexual dominant from a different country—I doubt he would have impacted my life so much. The universe has an uncanny way of giving us exactly what we need, when we need it, even if we don't know it at the time.

Certainly, I didn't always agree with Shane's ideas—like "devouring little dik-dik men." Nor was I ever fully sold on his concept and labeling of "alpha" and "beta" men. But he lured me into uncharted moral domain that ultimately helped me think for myself and ascertain what was right and true to me. My core beliefs were a bit expanded, and a lot reinforced: Although I discovered the merits of experiencing nonlove sex with different men, I didn't believe it was okay for someone to carry a dark agenda, like humiliating men for the sake of power. I believe one's intentions counted for a lot. And whether a sexual liaison transpired under the canopy of dominance and submission or traditional give-and-take pleasure, I believed that an attitude of harmlessness and respect should *always* prevail.

Still, I was disappointed. The sudden twist in events felt like a sick joke. We were so close to meeting and all the components had been in place: freedom to travel, mental connection, sexual intrigue, a lovely large penis . . .

How was I to know he'd want to stick it in my bum?

CHAPTER 20
THE DOM AND THE DRAGONFLY

WITH SHANE OUT OF THE picture, my man pool had officially dried up. Not even a prospect on the horizon. I looked straight into the void before me and asked myself: *Are you ready to stop this manic dating and get back to your old life? FINALLY?*

But I knew I wasn't, and sure enough, my inner Wild Woman stirred, restless, and offered up an emphatic *NO*.

Shane had left me unfulfilled—literally and figuratively. I had no clue how to reorient myself toward that land we'd been sailing to. How *does* one find a D/s relationship? And was I really seeking it, or was I merely curious? I forced myself to surf around the more "vanilla" dating site I was member to—where I'd met Chad, Brent, Adonis Boy, and countless other castaways—but I was bored. Same faces, same old sea. I was itching for something different, something *more* . . .

My trip to Vegas and the short-lived promise of a trip to New York had raised the bar a notch. I didn't just want romance and sex, I wanted travel. I wanted adventure. I wanted to pack my bags and fly off to meet an enticing new man in an exciting new city. I wanted to park Delaine the Ex-Wife and Mom at the airport and walk through the boarding gates with a carte blanche identity. I wanted to be free to express myself without the same self-imposed restrictions I faced at home.

What about the kids? I suddenly thought, feeling guilty and selfish. *How can I even think about leaving them? What if something terrible happens while I'm away?*

But I knew that was no way to live. I could be at the grocery store and something terrible could happen. And I knew my deeper, restless self wouldn't settle for staying put. I'd be a tiger in a cage, pacing my kitchen floor, only half present to the kids, unless I followed this personal journey to its end. Plus, I could plan my trips for the weekends the kids were with their dad. *Okay, Guilty Conscience, try again!*

What if you fall in love with a man who lives in a different city? Or worse, another country?

Good point! But I wasn't talking about love here. This wasn't about finding a replacement husband, nor even a boyfriend—*or a* friend with benefits. I just wanted to explore ME more.

Besides, Wild Woman chimed in mischievously, *why limit it to one man? Nobody has to know . . .*

Hmmm. She had a point.

Potential scenarios played out in my head. At home, I would have my own fulfilling and independent life—which included dating anyone I pleased—and the same rules would apply to my out-of-town lover. The difference would be that each month or so, we'd look forward to meeting for a couple of fun-filled days in one another's city. Maybe even in a third location. Like Vegas . . .

Perfect.

One guideline: I'd want them to be my age or older, and successful and independent. From my experiences with younger men, I definitely wanted wisdom and smarts over brawn and muscle.

I knew of only one place to find such men.

I cancelled my membership on the local dating site and logged on to the Sugar Daddy site with renewed interest. *Time to upgrade my profile and photos. Time to recast my fishing line into deeper waters.*

WHAT WERE THE chances? They seemed so slim that I figured it must be some kind of sign. Out of all the thousands of men on the millionaire dating site, I attracted another sexual dominant.

There was just *something* about the whole dominant/submissive thing that seized my attention. I chastised myself for my curiosity around it; why would I want to be "dominated" when I sought my own empowerment? That made no logical sense. I just exited a controlling marriage and a love affair that was heading down the same path. Was I subconsciously pursuing the same dynamic yet again?

But the pull was there. My body responded to it and I needed to learn more.

When John first messaged me, his photos immediately piqued my interest: He looked boyishly handsome, in a younger Harrison Ford kind of way. And as I read through his lengthy written profile, I grew increasingly impressed by how expressive he was. I gasped when I got to the very last sentence: "And by the way, I am a dom, as in D/s." As if it was an afterthought!

Right away I arranged to chat with him by phone; I had *lots* of questions. But unlike my first call with Shane, I felt no panicked need to write those questions down. And as our conversation gradually moved to D/s, I listened closely for any signs of danger or freakishness.

Immediately he explained that he (like Shane) was more interested in the mental side of D/s, though it "might" include some tactile elements, such as spanking, hair pulling, and using toys. "It really depends on what the submissive wants," he said. "People have this misconception that a submissive is vulnerable and weak and at the Dom's mercy. But that's completely wrong. A Dom never takes away. He only *builds.*"

A D/s relationship, in its truest form, is all about the submissive, he explained patiently. It's about *her* wants, *her* needs, *her* fantasies. Some of her desires may be conscious, but others may be locked in her subconscious. The Dom's job is to build a bond so strong with her that she feels safe enough, connected enough with him, to unleash her creativity and explore her innermost self. Through submission, she actually becomes empowered because she connects with her body, heart, and mind in much deeper ways.

"Trust. Honesty. Communication. And Respect," he said firmly. "Remember those four words. Those are the four pillars that a genuine D/s relationship is built upon. And until they are in place with any dom, *always* meet in a public place and *always* keep your clothes on," he warned, "because there are men out there who use D/s as a way to abuse women. They think sex is all about them, that they can take whatever they want. I've been active in the D/s lifestyle for the past fifteen years and I've seen enough and heard enough to know that subs have to be *very* careful. Otherwise, you can end up in the hospital."

Okay, now I was scared. *Hang up, hang up!* a voice shrieked in my head. *This is a sexual underground full of wackos. You're still WAY too naive to go here.*

Nonetheless, I kept talking to him. I appreciated the fact that he was warning me. And I liked that our conversation switched easily to other aspects of our lives: family, work, past relationships. Unlike Shane, who'd been secretive and much more about the sex, John seemed an open book. He talked about his family—his younger sister who was pursuing her dream to become a violinist in New York City, his widowed mom and divorced brother who were very active in the church community, and his fourteen-year-old nephew, who regularly dropped in to play his Wii and raid his fridge. I found his devotion very warming, and when I mentioned this, he replied: "I am a very loving and caring man, Delaine. I love and laugh and work and play just like everyone else. The only difference is that I'm also a dom. It's who I am and who I must continue to be. Once a person explores D/s, once he or she experiences the intensity of that connection, he can't go back to regular 'vanilla' relationships."

As our conversation progressed, I gazed over at my computer screen where my favorite profile photo of him sat open. Arms loosely at his sides, he was leaning back against a wall wearing dark jeans and a simple white T-shirt. His gaze was slightly off to the side of the camera lens, and a soft smile spread across his clean-shaven face. *He looks like the "man next door,"* I thought to myself, knowing that he lived in the suburbs. Then: *I sure wish a cute dom would move onto my street!*

I asked: "But since you're single, I assume you must get sexually frustrated sometimes. Do you have a friend with benefits somewhere to help you out? Don't you ever have one-night stands?"

"No," he stated matter-of-factly. "It's been over a year since my last relationship and since I've had sex. I'd rather take care of myself than pick up some woman at a bar. I'm not twenty-five years old anymore; I am in control of myself, my body, and my life. I choose to wait for the mental connection."

He then asked if I'd heard the term "subspace" before. When I told him I hadn't, he explained: "Subspace is the name given to the state that a submissive often goes into with her dom. Usually it happens after she's had multiple orgasms and her mind and body are on overload. It's kind of like being half-asleep, half-awake, yet it's euphoric and she can remain in that place for up to an hour—at least, from what I've experienced."

"And what do you do when she's off in subspace? Go have a coffee?" I asked, cheeky.

He ignored my flip tone. "I may exit the room, but only for a few minutes. It's my job to watch over her, stay close to her, and make sure she's okay."

"But don't *you* ever want to go into subspace?" I blurted.

"No. I'm a dominant. My pleasure comes from giving her what she wants and needs. My pleasure is derived from the connection I feel with my partner."

"I see," I answered weakly. But I really didn't see or understand at all. *You mean to tell me a dominant is someone whose goal and greatest pleasure is to explore and satisfy a woman's every sexual want and need? WHAT?* My body raced with excitement—this news couldn't get any better! But my brain was scanning for the loophole. Surely there had to be a catch. . . .

John, noting my long silence, gently asked, "What are you looking for Delaine?"

"I . . . I'm not really sure." He patiently sat on the line. "I've never been in a D/s relationship before, and I don't know if it's what I really want. But I do know I'm drawn to it, even more so now that I've talked to you about it," I admitted. "I do believe I have a submissive side to me. And I *do* want to explore it. My body totally responds to it—it shocks me, actually. But it scares me too," I went on. "There's so much I don't know. And from what you've told me, a real element of trust needs to be in place between the dom and sub. And I'm kind of lacking in the trust department."

He waited, his attentive silence coaxing me to talk. And so I told him about Robert's and Graham's betrayals. And it felt strange to tell my stories again out loud. On the one hand I felt removed from them, yet at the same time, a few silent tears fell while I spoke. John listened quietly until I finished.

"Good God," he finally said, exhaling loudly. "What a twisted story. And I have to say, though Graham sounds like a jerk, your ex is even worse. He sounds like a selfish little boy."

"Yes, he made some bad choices," I replied. "But he was younger than me and I just don't think he was ready to have three kids before the age of thirty. I changed a lot when I became a mother: I didn't want to party and get drunk anymore. He, on the other hand, did. I didn't think it was my place to tell him when or if he could go out at night, so I gave him his freedom. And the next morning, *if* he came home, I would usher the kids downstairs and try to keep them quiet so he could sleep it off until noon."

I continued: "Sometimes though, he never even came home—he crashed at a friend's place, which of course was his girlfriend's house. But I'd always been okay with him staying at a friend's place because he had a history of drinking and driving. At least this way I knew he was safe," I said, laughing dryly. "I didn't realize I was enabling his affair.

"Oh well," I sighed. "It's all water under the bridge now. It's all worked out for the best."

"Why are you defending him?"

"*Pardon?*"

"Why are you defending him?" He was irritated. "The man chose to abandon his wife and kids at night so he could go out, get drunk, and fuck other women. I don't care how hard he worked or how many days he worked out of town. He should have come home and risen up to his responsibilities as a husband and a father. It doesn't matter if he was younger than you, he chose to have children. He chose to have sex with you, get you pregnant, and bring them into this world. But instead of acting like a real man and taking care of his family, he was more interested in getting drunk and getting his rocks off."

The force of John's words caught me off guard. *I mustn't be describing this fairly*, I thought to myself.

"Remember John, you're only hearing my side of the story. I'm sure I was an imperfect wife in many ways. I contributed to the demise of my marriage, too."

"Of course you weren't the perfect wife. There's no such thing," he answered curtly. "But the bottom line is that when things got tough, when life was demanding and you and your kids needed him most, he only thought about himself."

He exhaled long again.

"Sorry to be so upfront, Delaine," he said more gently. "I know it's none of my business and I'm inserting my opinion without your asking. I'm ferociously protective of the people I love—I would do anything for them. And when I hear stories about men putting their cocks before the needs of their wives and kids, it repulses me."

Later on that night, as I lay in bed trying to sleep, John's comments around Robert kept jabbing me awake. I knew he was just an outsider, a stranger, looking in on my marriage for but a few minutes. But his judgment of Robert was so absolute. And I wondered: *Was his summation right? And did it even matter anymore?*

For a few brief minutes, I allowed myself to go back in time to revisit my marriage. It didn't take long for the old feelings of hurt and anger to resurface. I knew that dwelling there would only suck me in and downward, so I quickly fast-forwarded to the now.

But John's vehement words wouldn't let go. Why *do* I defend Robert and make excuses for his behavior?

I didn't think I was "defending" Robert so much as trying to be fair. We've all heard, after all, that "relationships are complicated things" and "the truth lies somewhere in between two people's stories." In essence, I was trying to view and speak of our history from a place of empathy and objectivity. That required I assume culpability for the role I played in its failure; to balance the scales, so-to-speak. I didn't think that should be perceived as "weakness." I think it was a very female way to perceive the world, for better or worse.

After all, we'd both lost: Our family was torn apart, and the wounds we each carried were real.

Over the next two weeks, John and I continued to talk every night by phone after I put the kids to bed. It felt strange, sometimes, going from snuggling with my bath-fresh babies, reading *Goodnight Moon* or *Where the Wild Things Are,* to then crossing into my own *Wild Things* territory soon after they fell into slumber. But it felt right, this distinction between my Mother Self and my Adult Self. *I was finally getting it* . . . I thought, feeling my equilibrium shift more to center. *It's okay to be a woman, too.*

Each conversation we shared was as lengthy and open as the first. An intense yet warm connection was developing between us; I'd dare to even call it a "special friendship." Would we ever go further? I wasn't sure. He never talked as if he was *my* dom. He referred to D/s in the third person. He never made any suggestion of us meeting, nor did he ever attempt to have phone sex with me. He just seemed to want to get to know me.

And I was letting him in.

IN KEEPING WITH my "date more than one man at a time" decision, I also started talking to Lornce, a successful businessman and entrepreneur. His energy was the polar opposite of John's. He was as excitable and distractible as John was calm and intense. I inevitably found myself smiling after our whirlwind phone conversations. There was never time to get "deep" with Lornce; his other line was always beeping or he was rushing to his next appointment somewhere in San Francisco. Still, his flitting, touch-base phone calls were most charming: "Hi beautiful!" he'd pipe into the line, when he'd burst briefly into my day. "Just saying a quick hello. Are you conquering the world? Shaping your kiddies into little Einsteins? Give that pretty ass of yours a pat! Ciao, gotta run!"

I felt his presence like the fleeting dance of a dragonfly: surprising, delightful, then . . . "outta here."

Lornce sent me a picture soon after we'd made contact—just his face. I'd studied it, trying not to be judgmental. He was pushing fifty and losing his hair, laugh lines and bags decorated his eyes, and his lips were thinning. As Hali put it, "He looks like your typical middle-aged man."

The truth was, had I met a man like Lornce locally, I highly doubt I'd have dated him. For the role of "out-of-town friend/lover," however, he merited consideration. More importantly, I found his intelligence very attractive (though he talked a mile a minute), and I enjoyed his silliness and the ease with which he laughed. I felt very unthreatened by him. Like he would enhance my world but not rock it.

Still, the physical attraction concerned me. I'd never been intimate with a much older man before, and I'd become accustomed to hunky younger men. What if he looked closer in age to my dad? *Ewww.* Then again, maybe his age and experience would make him a more attentive lover. *Hmm,* I'd hate to get his hopes up and fly down to San Francisco only to reject him.

For yes, he was already pushing to meet. He'd eagerly given me his personal info and I'd not only Googled him, but I'd paid for a background check on him through an online service; everything appeared fine. My next concern, however, was that I'd feel guilted or pressured into having sex with him; eventually, I came right out and told him so.

He was totally understanding. "If, when we meet, you decide you only want to be friends, I'm perfectly alright with that. I know this whole situation requires a huge leap of faith on your part and I respect that. *My* only concern is that I'll like you too much," he added, laughing. "You seem very real and honest. Plus, you're smart and sexy-as-hell. So . . . if it'll set your mind at ease, I'll fly *there* to meet you."

Thus it was arranged: my Dragonfly Man would be fluttering first class to Calgary ten days hence, in mid-December. Snow would be thick. Travel uncertain. Obviously, he was a man of action; a man who wasn't afraid to take risks, not just in business, but in life. And what wasn't to like about a man going the extra two thousand miles for me?

TWO DAYS LATER, I received an urgent phone call from Hali. "Tara's flying in tonight at seven thirty. She found out Matt's having an affair."

Oh dear God. Hali and I both knew what had to be done: Tara needed to be cocooned by her best friends.

As soon as my kids were asleep in the sitter's care, I grabbed my overnight bag and jumped in the car. Driving across the city, I thought back to the last time I'd seen Tara: We were at Black Cloud Brian's comedy club and her beautiful blue eyes had looked so *sad.*

I had expected this moment to arrive in one shape or another. Their marriage had been locked in a state of inertia for ages. I'd sensed something "big" would propel them into motion again, upward or down. I just wish she'd been the one to find a lover, not him. Now she had to deal with his betrayal—for the second time—and go through the painful divorce process. My heart wept for her, knowing the utter devastation she was feeling right now.

As I walked into Hali's house, I saw Tara and greeted her immediately with a long tender hug. She was already in her pajamas and her long blond hair was pulled back in a ponytail. Her eyes were puffy from crying, her face worn and tired. Shock had done its number on her.

"Thanks for coming, Delaine," she said in my ear, squeezing me back.

Hali came in from the kitchen. "Hey girl, thanks for getting here so fast," she said warmly. She was carrying a bottle of wine and three glasses by their stems. "Since you're both spending the night, let's go get cozy upstairs. Get our jammies on, pretend we're nine or something, kay?"

As we headed upstairs, me in the rear, Hali called back.

"Delaine, maybe you should grab another bottle from the fridge. Fuck having to leave our cozy room, right?"

Tara laughed and I obliged.

Back upstairs, I quickly donned my Super Girl attire, wondering when I'd last had a "sleepover" at a girlfriend's house. University? That was more a case of me passing out on someone's couch. When then? Fifth grade? My mind flashed with memories of pillow fights, sleeping bags, and ghost stories. Hardly on tonight's agenda.

The girls were sprawled across Hail's king-size bed, already immersed in conversation, when I rejoined them. I quickly found an open space and listened in. Hali, who'd become an overnight expert in the legalities of divorce, was answering Tara's quick-fire questions about the nuances of separation and divorce, reassuring her of her rights.

So it's come to this, I thought with empathy. *Oh my dear, we're here for you.*

Finally, Tara turned to me and told me her story. She explained that a few days ago, Matt had said he was going away on business. And though he commonly traveled for work, this time her spider senses wouldn't stop tingling. On impulse, she'd hired a private investigator and had him trailed. The evidence delivered to her was 100 percent conclusive: Matt was on romantic sojourn with a colleague from work.

Then came the dramatic confrontation. Tara, though reeling with shock and hurt, donned a brave face and calmly demanded an explanation. But none was forthcoming. Matt was furious she'd had him followed and couldn't get over it. He went on the offensive, yelling, name-calling, lying, blaming, while Tara stood there shell-shocked and numb.

"I could feel myself withdrawing deeper and deeper into myself," she said numbly. "I couldn't believe *he* was attacking *me*.

I couldn't believe this selfish, angry, unselfaware man was my husband. I mean, I knew he was like that. But it was like, 'Tara, why are you fighting for this guy?' *So what* if you've been married for fifteen years and have two kids together. You don't have to spend the rest of your life being treated this way."

Hali and I nodded somberly as Tara reached for a tissue and dabbed her eyes. Suddenly, out of the corner of her mouth she muttered, "Well, at least now I know he's not gay!" Hali and I burst out laughing. "Seriously!" she said now grinning. "Considering how little he wanted sex, I wouldn't have been surprised if I'd found out he was with a man." And laughter relieved our heavy hearts for a moment.

All these years we'd been friends, I'd assumed our married sex lives were so different—she'd always wanted much more sex from her husband, whereas I'd wanted much less. But beneath the surface we suffered the same wound, it had just been inflicted through opposite means: her body ached from the suppression of her need, my body ached with my need to suppress. Ultimately, both of us were being disempowered by our sex lives. Even though we tried to deny it and convince ourselves otherwise, some chunk of our souls had been slowly rotting away. Rejected. Dejected. Unheard. And I wondered how long we'd have let it go on had our partners not had affairs: Would we ever have found the courage to leave on our own? Or would our sense of duty, our fears and insecurities, have held us hostage?

Isn't every woman presented with big personal life choices at one time or another? Whether it's to have a child, quit a job, move to a new city, get married, or even have an affair. And if she finds herself standing at the critical fork of "Stay Married or Get Divorced," will she feel cornered by the scrum of her own fears, by the voices and opinions of other people and society? I know I was. So what do we do? Do we hang around at the crossroads for the rest of our days, too afraid to commit to one path or another, and resign ourselves to thinking that a "full life" is never our destiny? Or, whether it's months or years in the making, will we choose a path—make a choice and not just commit to it, but take action to either change it into what we *do* want or start anew on our own? Only we can decide when or if we're ready to make that decision, to face the fears and pitfalls and hurtles that we'll be confronted with. Without trying, ours souls would cease to grow.

Now, in the warm, cozy setting of Hali's bedroom, with the bluesy music of Norah Jones playing over the stereo, Hali and I tended to our bewildered friend as she adjusted to her new surroundings: the dreaded "Wilderness." We knew her journey ahead would be arduous and full of internal and external obstacles, but for tonight, we, her fellow warriors, would bear her weight as she took her first few shaky steps.

As our evening progressed, I inevitably found myself looking back over my shoulder to my own personal D-Day—the day the Graham Bomb exploded. And that's when it struck me: I had come a long way. For some reason, I'd envisioned myself like an anchored boat at sea, rocking about, but not really going anywhere. But in reaching out to help Tara, I was given a new yardstick, a new perspective, on just how far I'd come. I was a survivor. A Warrior. A Woman with a History, who would one day let it flow behind her like a colorful silk scarf.

And even though I still felt bruised, even though I knew I was still a work in progress, sitting there in Hali's room with my best friends I became aware of another feeling stirring in my body: excitement. For I was *changing*. I felt it—viscerally, emotionally, psychologically—I was becoming stronger, a bit wiser, a bit more confident; a broader, fuller me was awakening beneath the crevices left behind by the destruction. Who might she become? How will she evolve? Her field of dreams was unknown, yet vast, her potential and possibilities still to be discovered. But one thing was clear: She was rousing.

As I looked over at Hali, I saw many of my own thoughts reflected in her eyes. This night wasn't just about Tara: There was learning in it for us all. Hali and I weren't meant to "save" Tara or expedite her journey. We were meant to offer her hope; we were half-lit beacons reminding her to have faith in herself and a bigger plan for her life. And as we affirmed Tara's belief in herself, we were further reinforcing our own.

And so it was that I experienced my first sleepover in more than twenty-five years. But it was special to me in a different way than those of my childhood. For what did we do? We talked, we shared, and we learned from each other's stories. We drank wine, read aloud passages from books, and brushed each other's hair. We got silly, we got emotional, we got recharged.

For one full night, three grown women were as adoring and intimate as young sisters. And when we finally laid down to sleep, feet touching, on Hali's giant king-size bed, it felt perfectly right. Our togetherness, our solidarity, made the world outside and its big, adult problems fade away.

CHAPTER 21
INTRODUCTIONS TO A NEW YEAR

As we slid into our booth at Chili's Restaurant and Bar, Tory and her younger sister, Shiloh, pelted me with questions.

"What happened with the Dragonfly Man?" fired Tory, before I'd even removed my winter jacket.

"Yeah, fill us in, girl!" chimed Shiloh.

Less than two weeks after my cathartic girl-night at Hali's, Lornce had followed through on his promise to visit. And I couldn't help but laugh: I obviously wasn't the only person who'd greatly anticipated our face-to-face meeting.

Feigning seriousness, Tory continued: "I hope you realize we're living vicariously through your dating adventures, Delaine. We're relying on you to educate us through your experiences. So tell us *everything*."

"Well . . ." I began, chuckling, as I bundled my jacket over the top of my purse beside me. "We had fun. And I *do* like him. It wasn't a love connection or anything. But yes, I do like him. So I'm going to see him again. I'm going to fly to San Francisco. Probably next month."

The girls giggled gleefully. "That's *so* cool."

I looked down at my hands, smirking from ear to ear. *Yeah*, I thought. *It is.*

The waitress arrived at our table and we cited off our usual order: Southwestern rolls and two quesadillas to split. Extra hot sauce and guacamole on the side.

Waitress gone, Tory quickly jumped in, elbows firmly planted on the table: "So . . . what did you do while he was here? Did you have fun? Did you have *sex*?"

My mind flashed to the Calgary arrivals gate terminal: me pacing, fidgeting, and making numerous trips to the ladies room. Oh the suspense! Every time the customs doors slid open and an unattractive older man passed through solo, I held my breath: *Please don't be Lornce, please don't be Lornce . . . Phew, he's hailing a taxi,* or *Phew, he's meeting his family.*

Then: *What the hell am I doing? This is CRAZY.* Then: *Every other normal person in this room is here to pick up a friend or loved one. But no-no-no, not THIS nutcase. I'm awaiting an online stranger from another country!*

Finally, I saw him come through the customs door. We immediately locked eyes and he smiled. So did I. He looked like his photo, only better: he stood tall, he didn't have a big belly (phew again), and he was wearing a cashmere sweater and slacks. I could see both confidence and playfulness in his stance as he walked straight over to me and locked me in a big hug.

"Wow, you're gorgeous!" he announced exuberantly over my back.

I laughed. "Hi Lornce, welcome to Canada . . ."

Grinning at the memory, I turned to my keyed-up girlfriends: "I picked him up at the airport at around six thirty. And then we jumped in my minivan and drove to a Thai restaurant for dinner."

"Was it awkward at first?" asked Tory.

"Actually, no. It felt perfectly comfortable. Maybe it's because I've been on so many first dates," I said, with a sly grin. "But I liked his energy right off the bat.

"We enjoyed a great dinner together and spent about three hours talking. He talks and thinks *really* fast, so I had to pay close attention to keep up with him. But he's really funny too. Mind you, I'm sure it helped that I had a couple glasses of wine."

"And *then*?" asked Tory.

"Give us the juice!" squealed Shiloh.

I laughed. "And *then* he drove my minivan to the hotel—because I couldn't drive. We drank some more wine and talked up in his room. *And . . .*" I knew they were dying for me to get there, so I added with relish, laughing, ". . . then we had *sex.*"

They were literally on the edge of their seats.

"And how was it?" Eyes wide, vicarious.

Hmmm, how to answer. I thought for a moment. "It was good," I said, with reservation, "but it wasn't fantastic." Then thinking I may have downplayed it too much, because it really *wasn't* bad, I quickly added, "But it was good, don't get me wrong."

"Did it feel strange to be with an older man after being with such yummy younger guys?" asked Tory, taking a sip of her diet coke.

"Not really," I answered honestly. "It's hard to explain. I wasn't overwhelmed with desire when I *looked* at him, but I was attracted to his energy and his personality; he was fun and easy to be around. So when it came down to sex, age really didn't seem to matter—the body parts were the same!" I said laughing.

"Did you find him more attentive than the younger guys?" asked Shiloh. "Because that's what they always say about older men."

I paused for a moment, remembering our foreplay. "No, I can't say he was any more attentive . . . or unusually highly skilled, for that matter. No doubt, he was concerned with my pleasure, and he wanted me to orgasm before he did. Plus, he had surprisingly good stamina—which I made great use of." I gave them a wink. "But overall, the sex was very vanilla and well . . . average. But he was lovely to cuddle and chat with afterwards."

"Hm," said Tory, leaning back. I sensed she had hoped for something juicier. I sipped my water and shrugged my shoulders.

"Oh! But I gotta tell ya," I suddenly added, a memory bursting to come out. "When we started messing around and clothes were coming off, I had to laugh—the guy had on two pairs of long underwear."

"*What?*" laughed Tory. "It wasn't even that cold out!"

"Yeah, well, I guess some Americans really do believe we live in the Arctic up here.

"Anyway, the next morning we went for breakfast, had some more good conversation. Then I drove him back to the airport to catch his flight. We kept it short and sweet; we planned it that way in case we didn't like each other. We'll spend more time together in San Francisco."

"You seem pretty relaxed about the whole thing," said Tory thoughtfully.

I shrugged. "If I wasn't talking to John, too—the dom—I'd probably get more wrapped up in it."

"Is the 'dom guy' planning to come here too?" asked Shiloh.

I sighed. "No, not at this point. I'm not sure *what* we're doing . . ."

When it came to talking about John, I didn't even know where to start. We'd already spent over thirty-six hours talking over the phone. And he was teaching me so many new things—about D/s . . . life . . . even myself.

Certainly, we sometimes discussed dominance and submission, but it was always in a mentor/student-like way. He seemed focused on helping me understand the D/s lifestyle and my submissive side, but not actually meeting. That being said, erotic tension often permeated our conversations. And I immediately connected with his voice as soon as I picked up the phone; I looked forward to them.

One of the things I found captivating about John was that there was no separating John the Man from John the Dom. It was simply part of who he was: Strong. Calm. Intuitive. When I spoke with him, I could *feel* him listening to me; reading me. He heard not only what I was saying, but what I *wasn't* saying. We constantly talked about me—my past, my feelings, my dreams, my sexuality. I felt like he was trying to figure out my mind, not because he had an agenda, but because he genuinely cared. I felt no pressure, no expectations. He seemed to want me to understand myself. He kept reiterating: "A dom never takes away, Delaine. He only *builds*." And he was doing just that: I always felt uplifted after talking to him. Never cut-off or burdened or drained, like when I was married to Robert. Not only were my conversations with John liberating, they affirmed to me that my voice did count; that I was worth listening to; and that this was how couples could and should feel when they communicated. So I was filing this information away as reference for my next serious relationship. Because I didn't deserve to be any-one's emotional punching bag. And I now understood that if a man took out his boxing gloves, I could simply choose to walk away.

I looked at Tory and Shiloh across the table. I exhaled loudly. "A part of me worries that you guys think this D/s stuff is really wacked and so am I for being interested in it."

"No!" Tory said quickly. "I don't think you're wacked at all. I just don't know much about D/s beyond what you've told me."

"I'm not interested in any of the freaky sadomasochistic stuff," I reassured. "I envision it more like the movie *9 1/2 Weeks* . . .

The girls were quiet, all ears, patiently waiting for more.

"Have you ever imagined what it would be like to have your husband pin your arms against the wall, calmly tell you you're going to do whatever he wants, and then proceed to have his way with you in whatever way he chose? Or can you imagine being out to dinner with him, and as you sit next to him drinking wine, he suddenly leans over and whispers in your ear a detailed sample of how he's going to enjoy you later? Wouldn't that totally turn you on and leave you anticipating what was to come?"

"Absolutely!" said Tory. "Those scenarios are totally arousing. I think most women secretly wish that would happen. But I know if *my* husband did it, I would burst out laughing. Seriously! He would be so awkward; it would be wayyyy outside his comfort zone."

I laughed. "OK . . . but a part of you can imagine that being 'submissive' in this respect would be a turn-on?"

"For sure," Tory replied, and Shiloh nodded her head vehemently.

"John told me that from a neuropsychological perspective, it makes sense for women to have a submissive side.

"Imagine the two main parts of the human brain," I said, using my hands to demonstrate. "Down here you have the lower brain and up here is the upper brain. John said the lower brain is our 'old' brain—we've had it since the beginning of time and throughout evolution. It's where our instinctive, primitive thinking lies, like the fight or flight response, or the biological urge to have sex and reproduce.

"To understand how our lower brain functions, you simply need look to other less-evolved primates. Like gorillas, for example. One of the behaviors you'll observe amongst female gorillas is their jockeying to win the 'alpha males' in the pack. The females prefer to associate with the stronger, more dominant gorillas. They *want* to submit to an alpha, knowing that he improves their chances of survival. It's about safety, protection, and well, having his babies.

"Today," I said, with a deep breath, "this same lower brain activity is still active in the *human* female brain. The difference with our species is that we also have this evolved *upper part* of our brains." I referred to my air drawing with my hand again. "The upper brain is where we store our values and beliefs and morals, which have been compiled through social conditioning; for example: our family, our work environment, our community, etcetera. As women of Western culture, our social conditioning teaches us the *exact opposite* thinking to our primitive brain: that we are men's equals, that submission in any form is a 'bad' thing, and that we can be as strong and dominant as men are—which is true in most respects. *But*," I added, pausing, "What sometimes happens is that the two parts of a woman's brain are at war. She knows she is an independent, self-sufficient person, capable of forging and managing her own life. Yet secretly or subconsciously, she may dream or fantasize about submitting to a man sexually or otherwise, all the while berating herself for doing so because she judges her thoughts as weak, clingy, or abnormal."

Tory and Shiloh were staring at me wide-eyed. I asked, "Did what I just said make any sense?"

"Yes," said Tory.

"I think so," smiled Shiloh. "It's fascinating!"

A moment of silence. Then Tory blurted, "Why do I suddenly feel like I don't know squat about sex? I'm thirty-eight years old for God's sake, I thought I knew so much!"

I smiled and nodded my head. "Believe me, my friend, I know that feeling all too well . . ."

I HUNG UP the phone with John the Dom and looked at the clock: 12:25 AM. A New Year was officially underway. And there I sat—alone, the kids upstairs in bed, watching the silent hand go around.

I wasn't sad. I actually felt very content; but alert too, as if I was waiting for something to happen. Like the wall was about to open up and suck me into a New Year.

But nothing changed. The room remained still. My cat stretched.

I laid back on my couch and stared at the ceiling. *I wonder if*

Hali and the rest of the girls are having fun. Almost all of my closest girlfriends were attending the same house party. I'd declined. I just wasn't in the mood; I felt like being quiet and spending the evening with my kids. Besides, I knew this party was mainly being attended by couples—including Hali and her new *boyfriend*.

Yup. Hali had a new man: Bobby. Three weeks now, and she was over the moon. He'd tracked her down on Facebook, of all places; they'd attended the same high school. And they were totally smitten with each other.

"He seems to be everything I want in a partner," Hali gushed, when she told me. "He's communicative and generous and family focused and so 'everything' that Paul wasn't . . ."

I was genuinely happy for Hali, but I found it ironic that I was less interested in "serious" now than I was eight months ago when I first started dating. God, I was so panicked to find a replacement partner back then! I'm not embarrassed by it—I was scared to death, hurting like hell, and thought "serious" was what I needed. But the universe gave me what I *really* needed: a multitude of unusual dating and sexual experiences that helped me further understand my body and my Self. It was an objective I never would have considered, if asked back then.

Still, some part of me ached to find love right away. But the wiser, postdivorce Delaine I was becoming cradled it to rest, soothing that longing like a child who didn't know any better. For given the depth of my wounds, given the healing and self-discovery I'd yet to master, I intuitively knew I was at risk of falling in love for the sake of the blissful feeling, not because it was real, true, or what was best for me. No—I didn't need a hero, a second party with broad shoulders to step in and save me. I needed to stay focused on making myself stronger and more limber from the inside out, and trust that the universe would bring me who and what I needed, when I *really* needed it.

I *did* feel a tweak of sadness that Hali and I weren't "partners in crime" anymore. A part of me also felt kind of dropped—like a casual high school boyfriend—because suddenly all her time and energy were diverted to him, to them. But I knew she wasn't neglecting me intentionally or maliciously; she just desperately wanted and needed a stable, loving family life. If I were an abandoned woman with a six-month-old baby, I'd probably do the same. It was simply time for Hali and me to branch off on our own forks in the river. I knew she was ready. And deep in my bones, I sensed I was too.

So, while my girlfriends reveled in their partnerships tonight, old and new, I had reveled in my own—with my children. Earlier in the evening, the kids and I had bundled up in snowsuits and gone tobogganing in the dark, on a hillside aglow in bright flood lights. Their rosy-cheeked smiles and cries of "Let's go AGAIN!" had splashed in technicolor against the crisp, night air. And as I'd barreled down the hill, my arms and legs wrapped snuggly around their little bodies, I found myself hooting and laughing like I was a kid again.

Once home, after getting jammied up, we warmed up with hot chocolate and mini-marshmallows. Then came balloons and noisemakers, and we held a mock midnight countdown, all of us howling like a pack of happy wolves. And in finale, instead of reading them a story before I tucked them into bed, we'd held our first "sharing circle." We all sat down on the living room floor and took turns talking about what we were grateful for. My kids, given their tender ages, actually surprised me with the depth of their contributions: "I'm thankful for my brother and sister and great grandma and great grandpa and two grandmas and two grandmas and (insert full list of all relatives) . . . and all the love in this home," said my seven-year-old son most seriously.

My daughter laid her head on my lap to think about it, then

said: "I'm thankful for all the pretty flowers in our garden because they give Jax (our cat) a nice place to lie down."

"I'm thankful for my brain and hands so I can build with Lego!" said my middle child with gusto. "And one day I'll build skyscrapers that homeless people can live in!"

Around and around our ceremonial circle continued . . . until silliness overtook purpose and thanks was being giving for "being able to burp the alphabet." Laughing, I chased them into the bathroom to brush their teeth.

Now, with my three sweet babies in bed and me lying on my couch in my jammies, my thoughts drifted to my phone conversation with John the Dom . . . and the warmth in my heart spread down into my pelvis. Things between us had definitely progressed: As of Christmas Day, he officially became my dom.

Which meant two things: One, we were now looking into flights, hoping to meet within the next month or so, at the tail end of January or beginning of February; and second, he was training me to be his submissive. No, it didn't entail anything freaky, because at the end of day, one can only get as "freaky" with D/s as the submissive wants. And I had no interest in being tied from the ceiling, or wearing a dog collar or anal plugs for a month, or participating in threesomes or orgies, or being abused to the point of severe pain or bleeding. Nonetheless, in accepting that he was my dom, there were rules of protocol I needed to abide by in terms of my sexual conduct and behavior. For example, I was to call him "sir" when responding to his directives. Pretty basic, I know, but for some reason, this rule really irritated me. I quickly learned, however, that NOT saying sir meant "punishment."

One night, at the beginning of our call, he said, "I think I want you naked as I talk to you tonight. Get undressed right now and lie down on your bed . . ." And when I forgot to say "yes sir" and instead said, "'K, Bossman, give me a minute to get to my room, would ya?" it was reprimand time.

"Stop where you are right now and get on your knees," he ordered. "Get on your knees *right now.*" Shocked, I did as he said. "Now bow your chin, you may not look up, and spread your legs . . . Spread them *further.* Now, who's your dom?"

"You are."

"You are, *what?*

"You are, *sir.*"

"When you address me you will always call me sir, got it? Not doing so is extremely disrespectful and I will *not* tolerate your disrespect. Do you understand that?"

"Yes, sir."

"Now take off your clothes and get on your bed. You are NOT going to orgasm tonight, even though I know you want to, even though I'm going to bring you so close, not just once, but over and over again. Got it? Answer me!"

"Yes, sir!"

Lesson enjoyably learned.

For reasons beyond me, I found these new exchanges very erotic. Yes, a part of me was somewhat shocked and pissed at him to actually say such things aloud to me. But I also admired him for having the guts to do so and to say them with such confidence and power. The bottom line was, a part of me was thoroughly responding to and enjoying it. I knew his goal wasn't to demean me; it was to give me what I wanted, even though I didn't know what that was. It's like together, John and I were actors who were creating and performing our own stage play; but behind the curtain, I was the producer—the person with the vision—and he was the director, the person with creative know-how and experience. And the wildest thing to me was that nowhere in the script was there ever a scene that involved *him* masturbating. Nope—every single one was devoted to *my* sexual pleasure, *my* orgasms, or denial thereof. *Hell, if this is D/s, it isn't freaky, it's the best damn sex ever invented!* I thought jokingly.

In turn, however, he now said he "owned" all of my orgasms. Only he would decide when or if I played. Thus, if at some point during the day I wanted to masturbate, I had to first phone him and ask for his permission in a very specific way: *"John, may I please have your permission to play and masturbate for you?"* If I asked incorrectly—forget to say "please," for example—he'd say no. A few times he has said no to my request just because he could: "For your own good," he stated. And it made me *nuts*. But nuts in a *good* way. It made me want it more. I knew I could lie and masturbate anyway, but I felt that lying would break our trust connection, that it would rob me of something. For the intensity of denial was very erotic; deep down, I could feel my sexual energy boiling, bubbling, culminating. What might I pull from this wellspring of sexuality?

Beyond our phone calls, John also sometimes gave me "homework," which to me, was more like deep, mental foreplay; it made me think about him all day long. It didn't consist of me regurgitating information he'd taught me, so much as me independently doing research. For example, one day I mentioned that I'd bought my first ever piece of erotic artwork, for my bedroom: a large horizontal painting of a nude woman lying on her stomach. She was propped on her elbows, her back arched like a cobra, yet her chin was facing down. As John listened to me describe it, he suddenly said, "Take a picture of it and send it to me,"—which I did, right away that morning. All day long, my body tingled with anticipation for that night's phone call. What would he, my experienced "master" sense was hidden within my creative unconscious?

But instead, only I was to exhume and decipher its meaning. "Look at her Delaine," he said, his voice almost a whisper, as I sat on my bed looking up at her. "Look at her and let your imagination go. There is a reason you chose her, a reason you want her on your wall. Find it . . ."

For over a minute, I sat on the line in silence, trying to uncover the words, as my eyes and mind trailed along the length of her creamy skin, and melded into the rich browns and red of the background. To me, she appeared to be accessing something within her. It was there in the lengthiness of her tilted neck; there, in the earnest grip of her hands. She was still—motionless—almost draped in shadows . . . yet there was movement; she was mustering something soft and ferocious from within her body.

"She's rousing her passion," I murmured to John. "She feels the power of its energy . . . and she is both rising and aroused. But she's exploring it, savoring it, controlling it, *on her own*." I paused to fully feel my own words. They felt like they were coming from some unknown part of me.

I continued: "Any man looking at her would be tantalized—she's beautiful . . . she's soft . . . the lines and curves of her body are enticing. Before long, however, that man's desire would turn to envy; for he'd realize he isn't invited into her private world of surrender. He has nothing to do with the cause."

John remained quiet. I continued digesting what I'd discovered. Finally: "And why did you choose her, Delaine? Tell me."

"I chose this painting," I said, more to myself than him, "because I see myself in her. I, too, am rousing." And in that moment of realization, I felt almost orgasmic. I, like she, was on her own, in isolation, discovering and harnessing the power of an energy she'd never allowed to surface. It was bliss that came from discovery—bliss from realizing it came from within and bliss that no one could take it from me.

Conversations like this with John were deeply personal to me. More so even than the "D/s play" we had begun. And looking to the future, to when we'd meet in person, I hoped somehow the two would merge—the kink and the depth. How, I had no idea. But I felt confident he wouldn't push me too far or hurt me in any way. He would honor my limits, yet lead me to explore beyond my sexual boundaries.

I also knew that when we met in person, he'd physically discipline me, in ways I'd yet explored, if I was rude or acting up. He said he understood that when I was resistant, I was actually testing him. And he's right. I needed to know he was strong enough to handle me, physically and mentally; that he wouldn't just pretend or play games; that he was truly worthy of my submission.

But he said he would always win. He would always put me in my place. And the more he did, the more I would trust and open to him.

I did trust him. I'd searched for disconnects in our phone calls, turn offs or warnings. But there had been none. Only his growing interest and faith in me, and me in him.

John never asked me for my trust, nor did he pressure me for it in any way. It just evolved on its own, gradually and unthreateningly. And it felt good to feel it again—my entire chest actually felt warmer, like a rusty valve in my heart was functioning again.

I looked over at the clock. One in the morning. Nearly one hour into the New Year and all was still calm.

I remember lying on this exact same couch around the same time last year. I'd secretly hoped that Graham and I would spend it together. But no. He'd instead chosen to attend a small house party. Probably with his pregnant girlfriend. Nonetheless, he'd phoned me just after midnight and whispered, "I love you, Delaine. I wish you were here with me. Happy New Year, my love." I'd then lain here for an hour, alone, keeping company with my romantic dreams of us in the year ahead.

Wow, I thought, shaking my head. I'd had no idea what was around the corner.

What *would* this New Year have in store for me? I could sense the energy of the future all around me, a vast field of potential . . . and I planned to mine it for all it was worth.

CHAPTER 22

BOXED, BOUND, AND DELIVERED

I PRESSED MY NOSE AGAINST the airplane window and gazed down at the reddish-brown mountains and arid landscape below. It was really hitting me now (those weren't no snowcapped Alberta Rockies down there!): In less than half an hour I'd be in Orange County, California, where I'd finally meet Sir John the Dom.

Even though the past eight months had been filled with erotic adventure, flying solo to another country to explore D/s with a stranger I'd met online was further than I thought I'd ever go. I couldn't stop smiling; this weekend I was not Delaine the Stay-at-Home Mom, I was just Delaine the Woman, venturing into the unknown, an inquisitive soul open to—even *hungry* for—new experience.

The cards had fallen into place to make this meeting transpire. John would be here on business all week, and since Orange County was closer to me than his hometown of Miami, it seemed the perfect rendezvous point.

I'd never been to "The OC" before, though I did visit Disneyland when I was ten. *I've gone from meeting Mickey Mouse to meeting a Dominant,* I thought, grinning. Yes, this was definitely a grown-ups–only adventure. And from the tip of my head to the bottom of my high-heeled shoes, I felt more than ready.

John and I went over the ground rules numerous times before I booked my flight—for there were serious "what ifs" to consider. Like the possibility of no physical attraction in person. Or feeling pressured into something I didn't want to do.

"I've booked another room for you in case you decide you'd prefer your own," he promised. "My company has a block of rooms reserved for us, so it's not an issue." He then gave me the reservation code, which I later confirmed with the hotel's front desk.

"And what if I decide I don't want to have sex?" I asked honestly. "How do I know you won't pressure me?"

"I'm going into this with no expectations, Delaine. Worst-case scenario: We'll enjoy a lovely weekend together as friends. I won't even so much as hold your hand. I'll wait for *you* to come to *me*."

His last statement made me smile: Was he being a gentleman or using the power of suggestion?

"Oh—I should forewarn you of something," he suddenly added. "I'm shipping a box of 'supplies' to the hotel, just in case we do decide to play. I think it best I express-post it verses bringing it on the plane, in case I get searched." He chuckled. "It would raise a lot of questions."

"Supplies?" I asked, heart rate suddenly accelerating. "What kind of supplies?"

"Nothing crazy-unusual Delaine," he said vaguely. "Just a few toys I think you might enjoy in your introduction to D/s."

"Like what?" I blurted. I felt like a kid who was dying to open a present. I just about squealed with delight. "Oh *come on*—won't you at least tell me one thing?"

"No," he said firmly. "There's no need to at this point. But I will say, I think you'll be pleased with my selections." John knew all too well that my experience with "toys" was very limited; not for lack of curiosity, just lack of opportunity: Given the delicacy of, um, "competition" for my attention, I'd always figured a dildo was something the man should introduce into the bedroom, not me, and no man ever had. Thus, though I was in no way opposed to vibrators, they'd been relegated to being a "me" toy. As for bondage, I'd blindfolded and tied a guy up once while I was in university . . . but unfortunately, that was the scale of it. Hence, I knew John's decision to withhold the contents of the box from me was very deliberate. He was luring me in . . .

John and I also decided on an "out" or "safe" word for me—in the event sex *did* end up on our itinerary. This is a word I say aloud if an activity becomes too much and I want it to stop. "It has to be an unusual word, something you wouldn't normally say while having sex," he explained. "If I ever hear that word, I will immediately shut down the scene, no questions asked." The secret word we agreed upon was Shreddies—my choice. (What can I say, it's what I had for breakfast!)

Suddenly, the plane grumbled, wheels were hitting pavement. I'd landed. *This is it,* I thought. *I'm really here . . .* Gathering up my carryon, I followed the flow of passengers into the terminal. Business suits, laptops, blackberries, skiers, sun-seekers— I merged into the frenzied activity around me with heightened anticipation. We were all going somewhere, doing something, shifting out of our everyday lives—or back into them. It was surreal, exciting. On my way to baggage claim, I detoured to the restroom to freshen up and calm my bundled nerves. I examined myself in the full-length mirror. I'd wanted to look casual but sexy, so I'd worn my most flattering dark jeans with black strappy heels and a red blouse, topped off by my beige, three-quarter-length spring jacket, which came through the trip surprisingly free of wrinkles. I closely examined my face in the mirror: my blue eyes alert, no makeup smudges or dark circles; checked my nostrils (booger free!), and nothing stuck between my teeth. I stepped back and fluffed up my long curly hair. *Not bad, girl,* I thought, smiling at my reflection. *Now go get him!* I grabbed my purse and headed to the arrivals gate.

The security doors slid open and I walked through, looking around . . .

Right away I saw him. He was standing by himself, leaning casually against the wall, wearing Levis and a plain white T-shirt.

My heart sank.

Yeah.

It's not that John was ugly or creepy looking. For he wasn't. And he did resemble his pictures; there was no denying they were the same man. But on first impression, he didn't match what I'd blown him up to be, which no doubt was massively unrealistic: a Harrison Ford look-alike (or at least a close cousin), oozing the same sexy, controlled calm as Mickey Rourke in *9 1/2 Weeks*. The John approaching me did not exude sexy in his bootcut jeans and untucked T-shirt, and his blond hair looked unkempt and thinner than in his photos. He basically looked very average—like any other forty-something man, not the Super Dom of my imagination. He was shorter than I expected, too. I guess five foot ten is taller in Delaine's Fantasyland.

With these judgments wreaking havoc on my expectations, I smiled big as he walked up to greet me.

"Hi Delaine," he said, smiling warmly, his eyes bright with anticipation. "How was your flight?"

"It was good, *really* good!" I said overzealously, trying to mask my disappointment.

I didn't reach out to hug him *or* shake his hand.

"Come . . ." he said, eying me funny for one long second. "Let's get your bags."

Time passed in a hazy blur as we waited for and retrieved my luggage. I was polite and made pleasant small talk with him, but underneath, an internal war was raging. A part of me felt panicked and wanted to bolt; but of course, that wasn't a viable (or kind) option given the circumstances. I felt angry with myself: I should have known better, given my history with the online dating world, that photos and phone calls can be misleading. But most of all, I was disappointed and confused: Sex aside, did I even want to be in this man's company all weekend long?

I needed to compose myself. "John, could you please excuse me a sec while I freshen up in the ladies room?"

"Of course. Take your time," he replied. "I have to check on our car rental anyway; it's being delivered to the hotel later. So once you're done, meet me outside," he said, pointing to where cabs were queued up in line.

Inside the bathroom, I squeezed myself and luggage into a stall and stood there clenching my fists, *FUUUUUUUUUUCK! What the fuck am I going to do?*

Don't you think you're overreacting? a sensible part of me reasoned. *So he's not what you expected physically, so your initial meeting didn't play out how you imagined. This is a man you shared hours of conversation with—erotic conversation, too. And he's a really decent, caring man . . . remember? You haven't even given him a chance!*

I sighed and shook my head. It was true. I was being brutally judgmental. And melodramatic. And mean. The very least I could do was respect him enough to relax and enjoy our time together as friends.

Ten minutes later, I exited the bathroom and met John outside.

"Ready?" he asked, calmly, brow raised. I knew he didn't just mean to catch a cab.

"I am," I said firmly, this time with a genuine smile.

Who knows? I thought as I opened the door and slid in. *Maybe my attraction for him will grow.*

Luckily, the issue of "same room" or "separate rooms" was easily postponed. John's company was holding a postconference wrap up in the meeting room upstairs, with hors d'oeuvres and cocktails. "I really should make an appearance," he said, matter-of-factly. "Are you in the mood to socialize?"

"Sure!" I replied, enthusiastically.

"Good." He smiled slightly. "How about if we check your luggage at the front desk for now?"

"Great idea." I replied, knowing he'd deliberately bought me some "time."

For the next hour, John introduced me around a packed room abuzz with predominantly male conversation. His engineering colleagues, maybe thirty in total, were also wearing casual clothes—some in jeans, some even in shorts. "We decided to ban suits for the last day," he said lightly when I'd whispered it felt more like a barbecue than a business meeting, "It's been a long week and everyone's ready to cut loose."

Without even trying, I found myself easily enjoying myself. The fact that I was Canadian spawned lots of questions and jokes; small talk flowed easily. John behaved like a total gentleman—making sure I was never alone, yet not smothering me and giving me space to socialize. Nor did he ever touch me. Not even so much as to guide me by the elbow. I watched John periodically out of the corner of my eye as he mingled. I couldn't help but notice how enrapt his colleagues were when he spoke; that he drew them in; that he carried an air of respect and power. Even in a group of men that looked like they could be hanging out at the beach, he was clearly the alpha in this room. Not that he was boisterous or domineering—rather, he spoke little but meant what he said. And he listened a lot. I liked that. I liked watching him listen. How his face remained calm. How his eyes took people in. How no one else here knew they were talking to a dom. Watching him, I could now imagine what he'd looked like all the many nights we'd spoken over the phone; I could attach a real life visual to his voice. And I found myself wondering about and imagining "other" things about this man—sexual things . . . unexplored things.

John the Dom of my imagination was yielding to John the Dom the real man.

UP IN OUR hotel room, I finished getting ready for dinner and sat on the end of the bed, waiting, while John finished preparing in the privacy of the bathroom. I had changed into a knee-length, royal blue dress and high-heeled sandals, and I felt pretty—though a bit self-conscious about my Canadian glow. As I stretched my right leg out to assess its whiteness and examine my painted toes, my depth perception shifted: Just behind my big toe lay the still-sealed toy box.

John came into the room dressed and clean-shaven, the light smell of cologne moving with him. My stomach fluttered immediately: He was wearing a sophisticated yet casual black suit jacket, clearly tailored, and pressed khakis. His body looked strong and fit under his clothes. I suddenly found him very attractive.

"You look beautiful," he said, giving me a smile of genuine appraisal.

I smiled back, a little coy. "Thank you, John. You look very fine yourself."

"Are you ready to go?" he asked, as he grabbed his wallet and car keys off the dresser; our Cadillac El Dorado had been delivered to the hotel as arranged.

I remained sitting. "Almost . . ." I said softly.

He turned and looked at me, evenly—not surprised, not inquisitive, just expectant, patient.

"I'd like to see what's in the toy box."

Without replying, he walked to the box and began slicing his keys through the packing tape with strong even strokes. This man did *not* bumble. I sat perched on the edge of the bed, watching, listening, anticipating . . .

"First," he stated evenly, "we have bondage cuffs." He placed them beside me on the bed. I picked them up gently, hesitantly, feeling the heaviness and smoothness of the leather-covered steel. My body tensed with both fear and excitement.

"More bondage straps," I heard him say. An assortment of leather and metal was laid on the bed.

Deep breath. *Keep cool, Delaine.*

"And this—" he said, as he began unwrapping a longer black object with a leather handle, "is a flogger." He watched my eyes as he handed it to me. "It's soft, isn't it?"

"Yes," I half-whispered. I touched the strands of thick leather spilling from the handle. *So this is what a real flogger looks like.*

"And this—" he continued, "is a crop." He held up a thin, two-foot-long riding crop. "You know how this is used, right?" He gripped the handle and began walking around the room, flicking it. *Snap.* I flinched as he snapped at the air. *Snap- Snap- Snap.* Louder: SNAP! SNAP! SNAP!

Suddenly, a scene from *9 1/2 Weeks* flashed before me: Mickey Rourke and Kim Basinger were in a dimly lit store; he was testing various riding crops and snapping them in the air. She sat there watching him, smiling. *That movie really was about D/s!* I thought. *They just never showed him using it on her.*

Shivers of excitement raced up my spine. John snapped his crop one final time . . . then handed it to me. The handle was warm from his grip.

He proceeded to pull out seven more toys, all of which were packaged dildos and vibrators. They were literally of every shape, size, and color. Some were so realistic, they looked like molds of real penises—veins and all; others were smooth and phallic, curved, or with ridges; one had a base with so many buttons, it looked like a control panel. Others were small handheld vibrating "bullets," no bigger than my thumb. But they all shared one thing in common: These weren't bachelorette party favors—they all meant business.

He passed each one to me without comment, as if he were handing me groceries to put away.

"And that's everything I packed in my toy box," he said, matter-of-factly.

I looked around the toy-covered bedspread and slowly nodded my head. They were but inanimate objects—harmless, unthreatening, even kind of cute. But in the hands of John, they would become tools for my pleasure. How would he use them, how many would he try, which did I fear/desire for him to use most? As I sat alone with my thoughts, John suddenly reached toward me. My body immediately stiffened; *brace yourself, he's going to kiss you!*

But no . . . he was reaching for the toys. A faint smile played on his lips as he began returning them to the box.

"Are you okay with what you saw?" he asked quietly as he glanced at me and repacked.

I sat up taller and cleared my throat. "Yes. I think so."

"Nothing in here astonished you or disgusted you?"

"No. Not really."

Long pause. The last item disappeared into the box. "Shall we go for dinner then?" he asked, standing right in front of me.

"Yes, that would be nice," I said, laughing lightly. I moved to reach my hand out to him, assuming he would escort me . . .

But he'd already turned his back to me and was walking to the door.

I LEANED AGAINST the railing of the hotel balcony having a cigarette. Night had fallen on Orange County and soft city lights shimmered in the distance. Below, palm trees swayed in the wind, the sound of their collective rustling suddenly broken by a loud splash in the pool six floors down.

A man had dived in and was now swimming its length using clean, practiced strokes. *Good for you,* I thought. *You swim, I'll smoke.* I grinned and relaxed into the warm air. *This is so much better than the minus-twenty temperatures back home.*

Home . . . it felt so far away. I closed my eyes and imagined being in my children's rooms. Right now my babies would be fast asleep. I could see their sweet little bodies all snuggled up, their faces soft and angelic. *Mommy loves you,* I whispered to each of them, stroking their silky hair with my hand. *Mommy will be home in one more sleep, don't worry.*

I opened my eyes and forced myself back to the present. I dragged on my cigarette, trying to ground myself in my body; a body that was in a foreign city, in an unfamiliar room, with a virtual online stranger.

You shouldn't be here! A voice suddenly screamed inside my brain. *Your REAL life is a thousand miles away. Your REAL place is with your kids, your friends, your family. Go-home go-home go-home!*

But I shook it off. I would be back in those shoes within forty-eight hours. I had come here to step out of the ordinary, to become *more* of Delaine.

I looked over my shoulder into our hotel suite. John was standing ten feet away with his back to me, going through his briefcase. I watched his khaki pants crease as he shifted onto his other foot. His blond head was down, studying a document under the dim light of the desk lamp. He looked so focused, so completely unaware of my presence, so . . . *in control.*

I gazed back out into the night air, my shoulders tense beside my ears. For some reason that "self-control" of his irked me. Irked me and aroused me and pissed me off all at the same time. During our candlelit steak dinner tonight, I'd deliberately kept the conversation platonic: work, kids, fitness, health. I was waiting: waiting for him to bring up the toy box; to veer the conversation into the sexual realm; to "launch his seduction."

But he didn't. Not a word. And as hours passed and the server removed the final plates from our table, I found myself growing impatient; frustrated. I began baiting him harder, pulling out all my "womanly charms" to test that control. I made sure he had full viewing pleasure when I leaned back in my chair and slowly crossed and uncrossed my legs. I leaned over the table seductively, I used my eyes, I made suggestive comments and threw doors wide open in conversation.

But he didn't budge—not a flinch. He never even moved to touch me. Not that I didn't see desire in his eyes—it was there, steady and intense, through the flickering shadows of the candle-light. But it never decided his actions; it remained under the thumb of his control. I swore I saw flickers of amusement, too. *You can play all the cards you want, Delaine,* I felt him say to me. *I am your Dom.* You *will come to* me.

Now, as I watched John from the balcony as he rifled through his briefcase in the light of the desk lamp, I *knew* . . .

I knew it was time.

I closed the sliding doors behind me and reached up and dragged the heavy curtains shut. I walked across the room, feeling ready, emboldened . . . past the table of toys to where John was standing with his back to me.

I turned him around to face me, and moved in close. His hands remained at his sides, his right hand still clutching papers. He looked down at me with calm curiosity.

"I want to play John."

He held my gaze firmly, yet also looked thoughtful. "*Do* you?" he said quietly, as he placed the documents back in his briefcase.

Suddenly he reached around, grabbed a fistful of my hair,

and pulled me close to his face. "You think you're ready?" he said, more commanding.

I could only nod slightly; his grip on my hair was tight. Was I scared? No. Surprised by his sudden move? Yes. But I was game. Like entering a Haunted House at the carnival, I was more excited than afraid. I was saying yes to a *ride,* after all, one meant to entertain, thrill, and titillate—one that was designed for *my* pleasure and would see me through unscathed.

"Are you ready to do as you're told? Are you ready to give yourself to me?"

"Yes." I said again, with emphasis.

His intense green eyes studied my face. "You know I'll never hurt you. But you also understand that I will expect you to do as I say."

"Yes, John," I replied. But my eyes were sparkling, a smirk played upon my lips. I *wanted* to provoke him.

Hand tightening on the back of my head, he pushed me down on my knees and held me there firmly. "*What was that?* Get in the position, open your knees. *Now say it again.*"

"*Yes,* John (humble, head down). I'm ready to give myself to you."

"Good girl," he said quietly.

"BUT—" I looked up and giggled mischievously. "You're probably going to have to *make me.*"

Suddenly I was dragged on my knees across the room by the hair. Shocked, yet strangely aroused by the pain and force of his unexpected move, it took me a few seconds to realize we'd stopped. His hand still held me by the hair. I heard ruffling; the sound of cardboard—*He's digging into the toy box!* I realized, and I immediately began struggling and tearing at his hand with my nails. He yanked my hair so hard I cried out. "Stop that right now," he said through his teeth. Then the feel of leather around one wrist. Then the other. They were bound behind my back.

"Much better," he said with satisfaction. My hands wrestled

within the steely confines of the cuffs, seeking weakness or room for escape, as he stood looking down at me. "Now assume the position: Bow your head and spread your knees."

But I was not to be a willing prisoner; he had control of my arms, not my mind. "Fuck you," I seethed, glaring up at him.

"No, *you* will fuck me. You will fuck me exactly as I want," he stated evenly. "But first you need to learn some manners."

He pulled me to my feet by my hair and led me to the wall, where he pressed his chest against me hard. Without the use of my hands, I felt powerless and dwarfed by his size. I turned my head away, he was NOT going to kiss me: *If he even so much as tries, I'll bite him!* Instead, his voice was in my ear. "Now let's see if we can teach Delaine some manners." One of his hands held me in place by the shoulder while the other moved possessively under my dress. I wriggled my hips and squeezed my legs together, trying to block and evade his hand. Shots of pain—*he was pinching my thighs apart!* His hands claimed their territory, and the pleasure of his fingers was so great, I couldn't help but moan loudly.

His lips were beside my ear. "I know what you want, Delaine," he whispered forcefully. "You're so fucking wet I can feel you begging me to fuck you. But that's not going to happen; you're not going to cum any time soon. Not until you learn some manners."

His fingers moved harder. I needed to escape them; I needed to escape his voice. I thrashed my head from side to side as if to say no, but my body, despite my mental protests, was clearly saying yes. "Are you ready to assume the position?" I heard. "Are you ready to apologize for being mouthy?"

But before I could even answer him, I orgasmed hard and cried out. John immediately stepped back from me, looking down in surprise at his hand, which was soaked. "You are NOT to orgasm without my permission!" he growled. I closed my eyes feeling strangely content that I'd surprised him.

He spun me around to face the wall, roughly undid my cuffs, then turned me back round to face him. I didn't protest at all, my body was basking in postorgasm glow. I was quickly stripped: dress pulled over my head, panties yanked down in one swoop. Cuffs were being placed back on my wrists—this time locked in front of me. Hand between my shoulder blades, he half-guided half-pushed me over to the coffee table.

"Get on the table. On your knees," he ordered crisply.

I looked at him, wide eyed. A look that said, *Are you fucking kidding me asshole?*

"NOW."

As I gingerly climbed up on to the table, he walked over to the toy box. I stood up tall on my knees watching him, feeling acutely aware of my nakedness, yet also curious with anticipation. *What the hell was he going to do now?*

He walked back toward me and my eyes moved to his hands. He carried a pink dildo in one hand, his riding crop in the other. *Oh boy, here we go!*

He slapped the pink dildo down in front of my hips, suctioning it to the table. "Ride it," he ordered. "You're obviously dying for some cock."

My mouth was wide open in shock. *As if!*

He slapped my ass hard with his hand and I fell forward onto my hands. He crouched over and lifted my chin. "Next time I use the crop. Now climb onto it and fuck it. NOW."

I dragged my body forward and positioned my hips over it. He held it upright and pushed me down onto it hard. Pleasure shot through me; my body welcomed being filled. But as I slowly began moving my hips, my mind was racing to process the newness and strangeness of what was transpiring. I was masturbating, on a coffee table, naked, in front of a fully dressed man who had handcuffed my wrists. I was a freak performing in a freak show; an animal pulled in from the wild. Yet that wasn't true at all—I wasn't forced into captivity but had done so willingly. My spectator was an invited audience member, not some passerby. And the act I was performing, in all its rawness and obscenity, was natural and felt blissfully good.

John walked slowly around me as my stage show continued, periodically snapping his crop. "That's it, my little slut . . . Good girl, move that ass . . . *Mmm*, you love that dildo in your pussy."

Slowly, my self-consciousness yielded to the feelings of pleasure. And attached to that pleasure was a feeling of power. For in having John stand by and watch, but a witness to my personal sexual fulfillment, I felt like I was choosing the toy over him; like he could stand there and try and direct my actions as much as he wanted, but the only person privy to the mounting pleasure was me; it was *mine*.

I suddenly felt John's fingers on my clit. Oh my god, it felt so good. But he was reminding me he wasn't just a spectator. He was the Dom and in charge.

"Are you ready to apologize for being mouthy, Delaine?"

"*Mm-hmm*," I moaned, so close to orgasm . . .

He grabbed my hips, immobilizing them with both of his hands. "I asked, '*Are you ready to apologize for being mouthy?*'"

"Yes," I said faintly.

"Yes, *what?*"

"Yes, *sir*."

"And what are you sorry for?"

"I'm sorry for being mouthy, sir."

"Good," he said and released my hips. "Now get down off there. It's going to be a long time before you orgasm yet . . ."

JOHN'S FLIGHT HOME on Sunday departed earlier than mine, so I stood with his luggage at the hotel entrance as he drove the rental car around. We'd spent Saturday driving up and down the coast, stopping whenever we so desired to shop, dine, or walk along the beach. John was pleasant and easygoing but remained true to his calm, self-controlled personality. Only once did I see him get ruffled—when the car's GPS system was being wonky. But that made me giggle: It took a "she" in the guise of a computer to make him lose his cool.

Now, as John threw his luggage in the trunk, I watched him closely . . . tenderly. Time felt like it was slowing down so I could imprint these last moments in my long-term memory. Despite what might come across as John's rough handling to the uninitiated, the experience fostered a deeper intimacy and bond with him; a backdrop to our broader relationship, which had always been underscored by kindness, depth, and sincerity. He helped me grow. I adored him for that—and for being John the Dom, when I needed him to be.

He took me into his arms for a big hug. My eyes filled with tears, and I embraced him tightly, knowing this was the one and only time I'd ever see this wonderful man; for we'd arrived at the decision earlier this morning. This moment was not just goodbye for now, but forever.

It wasn't that we didn't click; in fact, we did very much. But the bottom line was that we both had lives in two different cities, in two different *countries*. The mere thought of what that type of relationship might entail over time—financially, emotionally, logistically—was just too much for me; too complicated. I wanted simple, I wanted free-flowing. No more upstream battles. And I didn't have room for that type of priority, not above my children. No, as much as he'd helped me grow, this was as far as we could go. It was time for me to stretch toward the sun myself. And I knew I could do it, on my own.

"Call me when you get home tonight so I know you got home safe, okay?" he said, as he wiped a tear from my cheek with his thumb.

"I will." I looked into his green eyes and saw his concern. "I'm okay," I laughed. "I'm just deeply grateful for everything we've shared this weekend. And prior to it. Thank you, John. Thank you."

He pulled me into another strong embrace. "You're an amazing woman, Delaine," he murmured.

Two minutes later, he and the rental car were gone.

Back up in our hotel suite, I lay down on the bed and looked around. It felt strange without him here. So empty and quiet. The weekend had gone by so fast: forty-eight hours, vanished—like a dream.

But I could feel his presence, the energy of our togetherness, lingering everywhere in the room. I turned my face into my pillow; I could still smell him on it. I smoothed my hand across the sheets, noticing a small stain from one of my many orgasms that the towels hadn't absorbed. *My God, he had made me climax!*—so intensely and so many times that my body had trembled for many minutes afterward. I couldn't even hold a thought in my head at that point. My body was so overloaded with ecstasy, my brain had just floated away. John had lain down beside me and smoothed my hair out of my face, caring for me, watching over me, protecting me. This heaven-like realm was what John had referred to as "subspace." I couldn't think, couldn't move, there was only light carrying me away . . . and lightness.

All alone now, I rolled over onto my back and stared up at the white ceiling with a sigh.

Flash!—neurons, electrons, and protons swarmed into a memory: my throat angled sharply off the side of the bed, mouth full and gagging.

Flash!—eyes veiled in darkness, the soft strands of the flogger trailing the length of my body.

Flash!—John hissing from the side of the bed: *"Kick me? You think it's okay to KICK me?* He walked to the dresser and put something in his pocket. He turned and looked at me coldly. *I think you need to lie there tied up and rethink that. I'll be back later.*

Flash!—The sound of the hotel door clicking shut. Staring at the ceiling aghast: *Holy fuck, the asshole actually left me here!* Struggling to get free. Lying back in defeat. Arms beginning to ache. Praying the hotel maid didn't show up. Staring at the ceiling for what seemed like an hour . . .

My mental screen dissolved into the present: I was staring at the ceiling now by choice, not confinement; John was gone and I was alone. But my heart was pounding; my body remembered.

No doubt, much of what I experienced with John that weekend involved my being physically "forced." And my "need" to experience that was scary and weird to me—it seemed dark . . . twisted . . . *violent*. It was one thing to have accepted my "need" to be taken by men during vanilla sex these past months; the former Delaine of soft touches and gentle kisses had certainly expanded. But in bringing the concept of "being taken" to being physically and sexually forced, potentially even demeaned, I feared I was subconsciously taking the abuse I'd endured in my marriage to the next level.

But I now realized that my fear was misguided. The sexual and physical control John exerted over me actually empowered me, not stole my power. For our connection was first and foremost psychological—a battle of the minds. I'd needed John's control and self-control to force my assertiveness, something I never did when disempowered and belittled in my marriage; his knowledge, his creativity, his outstanding intuitive abilities helped direct that. The act of learning to submit forced me to assert myself enough that I felt confident and trusting enough to *willingly* submit, and for my gain not my loss. I had "submitted" to Robert against my will, and at great emotional cost, throughout my entire marriage. I didn't trust myself—or believe in myself enough—to take control. John was the foil to my passivity and mistrust. And in opening up to him, in allowing him to dominate me, I'd made him "earn me." Unlike Robert . . . who had "taken" from me for himself, sexually and emotionally.

So in the strangest of ways, the D/s relationship I shared with John—from our many phone calls right through to the scenes in our hotel room—had helped free me from the wounds of my marriage. The sex we'd shared in this room had been the final gateway—a passage through which I was able to learn to trust a man again and to claim the ecstasy and power of my sexual energy as my own.

As I lay in bed relishing the warmth of these revelations, I wondered how my weekend's sexual adventures would affect me once home in Calgary. I knew my exploration hadn't much changed me as *added* to me; I'd become *more* of Delaine. The woman I envisioned returning home carried herself with more confidence. She was in tune with her passion and creativity and saw the value in keeping those channels open. She had more faith in her body's intuition and no longer quashed it without listening. She felt freer and more capable of expressing her wants and needs, not just in bed but in life.

My mind returned to John, wondering if he'd already boarded his plane. He'd invested a great deal of time and energy in me, offering me the most tender and unselfish "friendship love" I'd ever known—*without* demanding anything in return, *without* taking anything away.

I rolled over on my side and curled peacefully into the fetal position. Once again, this body of mine, the house of my sexual energy, had initiated an adventure for me. And by choosing to listen to it instead of ignoring it or judging it, many other levels of learning had opened to me. It had guided me into the beauty of submission. It had guided me to John. And, ultimately, it had guided me to new heights of ecstasy that had required and enabled me to trust again.

CHAPTER 23

THE PRIMARY SHAREHOLDER OF MY HEART

I SMILED AS I REREAD the travel itinerary lying on my desk. In less than two weeks, I'd be flying to San Francisco to meet Lornce. And as I listened to the minus-thirty gale howling outside my office window, all I could think was, *Thank God!*

Six weeks had passed since my weekend with John. I'd come back reenergized about life, about myself. The experience had been transformative—not just sexually, but in the realm of the heart, too. I had bonded deeply with a man and resisted the urge to force more out of it than was meant. It showed that my scales were continuing to tip toward self-purpose and independence. *And* healing. Sure, I found myself missing the intimacy that grew out of our conversations, but I knew the relationship had run its course: I had learned everything I was meant to learn from him. And even on the occasional night when I awoke seized by anxiety over being a single parent of three kids—with all its attendant pressures—still, I felt the change in my bones. I knew I could withstand, even prevail in, a future on my own; I could become the architect of my own life, a feeling I'd never fully experienced. And somehow, flying off to see Dragonfly Lornce seemed a necessary part of the blueprint.

Suddenly the phone rang. *Who's calling this late?* I wondered. It was nearly midnight. For a brief second, I thought maybe it was John . . . Then Hali's number popped up. I quickly grabbed it, excited to tell her my travel news, but she had her own big news: "You'll never guess who showed up unannounced at my door tonight."

"Oh, no . . . Who?" I asked, but I had my suspicions.

"PAUL. He came over to tell me he still loves me. He wants to get back together."

Yep. I knew it, I thought as I clenched the phone and my teeth. As a bystander, I'd seen this shot being thrown out of left field. Hali, on the other hand, was knocked upside the head.

Not only that, but he'd arrived fully armed, offering words that every betrayed, abandoned (while pregnant!) woman aches to hear: "From the bottom of my heart, I'm sorry"; "I made a huge mistake"; "The problem was mine, not yours." Paul spoke earnestly, she said, words that caressed her heart and made her weep with *relief*—some part of her had always wondered, *Was I that horrible to be married to?*

But as usual, Paul's timing sucked. Over the last few months, Hali had developed pretty serious feelings for her boyfriend, Bobby. He seemed to be everything Hali wanted in a partner: He treated her with respect and kindness *and* seemed to be a real family man. Truly, the only problem she'd encountered with their relationship was that it seemed *too* perfect.

"I keep looking for signs that Bobby's putting on an act," she'd said countless times since they started dating. "Maybe he's just trying to impress me, right? But no matter where we are or who we're with, he's always the same guy. I even asked his sister and mom, 'Is he *always* like this?' And they said, 'Yup, this is just who he is.'"

With Paul's sudden about-face, Hali found herself at yet another crossroads: Should she move forward with Bobby, a man who was Paul's opposite, in a relationship that felt right on every level but was dangerously new? Or should she go back to her husband, the man she shared a history with, and try to revive their love and knit their family back together?

Half out of a sense of duty and half because she still had feelings for Paul, she went back to him.

"I just have to give him another try," she reiterated to me before saying goodnight. But as I put the phone down, I knew it was more to convince herself than me.

Very quickly, Hali found herself an emotional mess all over again. "I feel sick inside," she lamented to me on their first day of reuniting. "I keep having to remind myself why I'm doing this. I'm trying to convince myself I've made the right choice. But it *feels—so—WRONG.*"

The next day, I heard: "It's the same old thing, Delaine. We're two days into it and everything about us is a struggle. He *says* he's a changed man, that his family means everything to him. But already today, it was same-old, same-old. First, he was late coming home from work. Then, after eating by himself, he laid down on the couch while I took care of the kids and did everything else, because his day was just *that* busy, you know. Like mine wasn't."

The third day: "Most of our conversations are still about *him*—his pain, his being lost, him not being able to express himself. I don't think he's much further ahead than where he was a year and a half ago.

Four days in: "I can't help but wonder, 'Do I *really* still love him? *Is* he the man I want to share the rest of my life with?' I know I love him in a way, but those feelings are all jumbled up with other feelings: nostalgia, compassion, pity . . . I'm just not sure he could ever make me feel special again, Delaine. *Really,* after all we've been through, how could I ever feel *special?*"

The fifth day: "I'm not convinced he's here for the right reasons. He *says* he loves me, but is he really in love with *me*, or does he just want his old life back: the kids, the house, the family dream? I just feel like I'm part of the backdrop of some ideal he's looking for, you know?"

By the end of the first week, Hali was done.

"I know it sounds crazy to make a big decision like this within a week, but I've changed too much and he hasn't. He's just giving me too little too late. I want more than what Paul can ever give me, and I know it's out there because I've had a taste of it with Bobby. And even though I don't know where our relationship will end up, loving him and spending time with him is just so darn *easy*. It just *feels* right. Moment to moment, day to day, I feel happy. I feel like he loves me for me, not because we have kids together, not because we shared vows, but simply because of me."

Who could argue with that? Not me. Every ounce of Hali's intuition was telling her this was the best and right choice. Why waste another second of her life floundering at the crossroad?

FOUR DAYS LATER, wearing the same travel clothes I'd worn to see John—dark jeans and a beige three-quarter-length jacket—I caught a 6:00 AM flight to San Francisco, where freedom of expression was not just embraced but encouraged. And I intended to live up to that standard, because this time, nervousness didn't impinge on my excitement. Unlike with my trip to meet John in the OC, I'd already met Lornce and knew I'd enjoy his company—in *and* out of our hotel room. It was like a really cool second date: forty hours with a great guy in one of the most beautiful (and liberated) cities in the world. I had no roles weighing me down, no expectations, I was simply free to be me—a carte blanche identity.

But the week before my trip, I suffered a crisis of confidence. *How can you leave your kids yet again? How selfish are you?*

One of my greatest struggles to date had been the guilt and emotional estrangement I'd felt as a mother after the chaos of Robert and Graham. Emotionally, I was bankrupt, but I desperately wanted to be the mom my kids knew and deserved. In the beginning, my inertia was terrifying. There was a wall up between me and everything, including them. But I had done many things right by my children. Like ensuring they were shielded from the animosity between Robert and me during the separation: Even when I was fuming or in tears, I either masked my emotions or excused myself to the bathroom or my bedroom until I pulled myself together. And when my kids expressed their sadness or anxiety around our divorce, my feelings took a backseat, and I listened, empathized, and reassured. I never put their father down in their presence, and I put their needs first.

Something else I'd done right was to show up for my mommy job every day, no matter what. Sometimes more in body than in heart, but I was there, I was consistent, and my presence was known. Furthermore, when I needed help, I *asked* for it. And this was tough for me in the realm of parenting because I viewed that job as my primary responsibility, and in floundering, I felt "less-than." But I accepted the help of a stellar baby sitter and when I needed a break—or a date . . . or two—I called her. And I felt smart doing that, not selfish. Because what my children needed was a happy, healthy mom raising them—and loving them—and I could only do that by exploring and nurturing myself, which is where I'd been headed these last eleven months. My D-Day anniversary was approaching, and Lornce was my last great fling. So I knew I had to put aside my maternal guilt and embrace the moment. And I did.

MY DRAGONFLY MAN showed up at the arrivals gate wearing not only a big smile, but his figurative tour guide hat. "A true San Franciscan, born and bred, so eagerly at the *sexy* lady's service," he said with a bow. I laughed and grabbed his hand: *Let's go!*

First stop on the tour was Chinatown, where we blended into the bustling crowd of local vendors and tourists. Strolling along hand in hand with Lornce, I got just as much of a kick out of watching him as the people around us—he was like watching the song "Zip-a Dee-Doo-Da-Day" in human form. I don't think he'd have batted an eyelash if a bluebird landed on his shoulder. He approached everything with such enthusiasm—including lunch: "I want to take you somewhere special," he said excitedly. "It's my favorite restaurant—Greek food—and tourists don't know about it!" Once there, I agreed to let Lornce do all the ordering for us (in secret, away from our table). I laughed in surprise when seven dishes arrived at our table. "I want you to try them all!" he said, his hands in the air, with a smile stretched equally as wide. How couldn't I adore the gesture?

We strolled along the infamous Fisherman's Wharf, gobbled giant chocolate ice cream cones, and visited a lesser-known museum where we wore individual headsets explaining the Marie Antoinette exhibit. And from the other side of the room, as I watched Lornce examine a painting then dip his hands in his pockets and disappear around the corner, I thought: *"Zip-a Dee-Ya . . ."*

Whether we were shopping, taking photos, basking in the sunshine, or exploring the gay district, I took it all in with the curiosity and wonderment of a child. I felt so appreciative of everything—the sites, the people, the weather, the man next to me. *I am so lucky to be here!* I thought countless times.

I felt myself stretching out, emotionally *and* physically. I literally found myself twirling in the streets with my arms outstretched, while Lornce stood by grinning. It didn't matter that this was only a holiday. I was here and the moment was real, so there was no reason to close down the feelings. I felt free, vibrant, unrestrained by my past, my "titles"—ex-spouse, mother, lover, friend, *everything,* even my sex life and what anyone else thought of me. I felt beautiful, confident, and for the first time in ages, truly *joyful*. I allowed that joy to surface, I allowed myself to feel it, radiate it, *be* it. It wasn't just circumstantial, it wasn't just because I was with a man or because I was in a new city. It was my True Self, my true and right way of being, shining through. *She wasn't dead after all,* I thought elated. *She'd just needed time for her rebirth.*

Late in the evening of my last night there, Lornce and I playfully fell into bed, and I voraciously devoured every ounce of his incredible stamina. The experience was so different from John, and I marveled that my sensuality, desire, and pleasure could flower under such varied conditions. Where sex with John was serious and intense, sex with Lornce was passionate yet sweet; both "flavors" bore remarkable resemblance to the men themselves. It wasn't a matter of one flavor being "better" than the other: each was pleasurable and satisfying in its own way. But without a doubt, my experience with D/s had freed me, emotionally and physically, to enjoy more conventional sex with abandon. Not that sex with Lornce went beyond standard foreplay and a mix of regular sexual positions, but I flirted, teased, took and gave with ease; I'd ridden a dildo on a coffee table wearing cuffs after all; Wild Woman had been embodied and set free . . .

Afterward, as I stood brushing my hair in the bathroom, Lornce leaned in the doorway watching me with a big grin on his face. "Wow, you were so different this time, Delaine."

"What?" I laughed, stopping midstroke.

"No. *Really.* The sex we just had was unbelievable. I mean it was great the last time we were together, but this time you were—" He mock wiped his forehead with his hand. "*Phew.* Absolutely incredible."

I laughed again. "Thanks, Lornce," I said lightly, offering no attempt at explanation. A woman's entitled to her own secrets, after all.

Later in bed, I curled up naked on my side with Lornce spooned tightly around me. *What a long but glorious day*, I thought, nestling into my pillow. I quickly began drifting off to sleep, but the sound of Lornce's soft voice in my ear pulled me back: "You are truly a special woman, Delaine. I've never met anyone like you before. You're just so many things: smart, fun, great in bed, warm, loving, open-minded. You're so . . . multidimensional."

Shocked, I laid there with my eyes open, tasting, digesting his words.

From behind me, he continued: "You're really an amazing woman."

I squeezed his arms and words around me, their warmth filling my soul. "Thank you Lornce," I whispered. "Thank you."

The next day on my flight home, as I replayed our time together, smiling, I wondered if Lornce and I would ever see each other again. My sense was no; it was better if we didn't. He was open to having a love affair, and friendship was as far as I wanted it to go.

But it was more than that. It was a feeling under my skin that my time with Lornce was done. Sharing this weekend away with him was what I had needed to finally stand in and embrace my joy. I wasn't a "boring old lady" like Robert used to say to me when the kids were young. I was fun, I was dynamic and interesting, and not only could men enjoy my company, I could, too. And to my amazed delight, the propensity of my joy seemed greater now than before my life had exploded. Maybe it felt that way because it was a long time coming; or maybe the intense suffering I'd endured magnified it. All I know for sure was that I welcomed it with an open heart. And no more trips were required.

If I had had this kind of romantic experience at any other time of my life, my heart would have whisked me away. I'd have daydreamed about my lover and yearned for him in his absence. Heck, when I was younger, I'd pine over men after just one date.

I wondered: *How is it that I've become so grounded and, in a way, detached?* Fear of intimacy? But I knew that wasn't completely true, because I was warm and caring with Lornce, and I opened myself to John the Dom on more levels than I had with any man in my life, leaving myself fully vulnerable—physically, emotionally, psychologically. True intimacy requires absolute trust, and I gave that to John and Lornce. No, this sense of emotional liberation, I realized, came from finally knowing that I could be with a man, be my real self, and not *lose* myself in him. I could welcome and appreciate each unique man who entered my life without assuming he was a love connection. It was like a new window had opened inside my brain, one that reminded me to be practical—*sensible*—when it came to relationships; that I shouldn't label something a masterpiece just because its brushstrokes appealed to me.

As I sat on the plane flying home from San Francisco, I felt enlightened; like I was finally starting to make sense of how and why I'd loved . . . and lost. In many ways, my heart had been doomed from the start. And though I recognized that my romantic idealism and neediness were still a part of me, I knew they would no longer automatically dictate my choices.

I've become the primary shareholder of my heart, I thought, as I stared out the plane's window. And I felt my True North, in every way.

EPILOGUE

I STOOD BRUSHING MY TEETH in the bathroom mirror, wearing a fuchsia push-up bra and matching silk panties. Robert had unexpectedly taken the kids for the night and I was beautifying for a last-minute drink date.

With Hali.

The lingerie was just for me.

Smiling, I flicked on my blow-dryer, and my thoughts floated back over the last few weeks and what it had brought. Spring had once again exploded around me, yet instead of feeling frostbitten by the shock and aloneness, like last year, I welcomed her with an already warm heart. The one-year anniversary of my D-Day had already passed, and I didn't fall apart or wallow in glorified memories or burn sage to exorcise the spirits of old love. Nope. It wasn't as emotionally monumental as I'd expected it to be, but it was certainly cathartic. I am an absolute believer in Karma, and the universe pulled no punches in delivering up an ironic end to my year of heartbreak and ultimate liberation.

Though I'd often seen my friend Sara at school during the school year, we never discussed Graham, his lover Melissa, or their baby. Bringing them up felt inappropriate to me; *uncomfortable*. Melissa was her friend, after all, and I didn't want Sara to feel like my "spy." No, I felt it better to avoid one-on-one luncheons altogether and keep whatever conversation we did share focused on our kids and school. Squashing my curiosity wasn't too hard—my dating life had well-trained me to bite my tongue and keep things "private."

But on a windy night near the end of March, we ran into each other at community soccer tryouts. I found myself standing on the sidelines alone with her, watching our seven-year-olds vie for team placement. And it was there, as we stood shoulder to shoulder, the wind whipping our hair, that I suddenly heard her say: "I talked to Melissa the other day."

My body froze. *There it was.* I kept my eyes glued to the field, hidden behind sunglasses. "How's she doing?" I asked politely.

"Not good." She looked down and paused as she kicked her heel hard into the grass. "She wanted me to come over and see her and Graham's daughter. She's almost one year old now."

My eyes remained on the field, my entire body motionless. "But I didn't go over," she continued. "Frankly, it's just too messy a situation for me."

The sound of her sigh suddenly reminded me to move. I turned toward her, slowly nodding my head, encouraging her to continue. *Go on*, I thought. *I need to hear this. Please keep talking . . .*

The story was worse than I could have imagined. Graham's ex-wife found out about the affair, told Melissa's husband, who then discovered the baby wasn't his, they split up, and Melissa and her five children were now living in a boarding house. And Graham? He abandoned Melissa in her hour of need as well—like he had done with me when Robert and I had separated. Yet he had the audacity to ask for half custody of his daughter. *Still no balls . . . or a conscience.*

But what did I feel? Morbid satisfaction, perhaps. Certainly, empathy for the kids, the baby, the betrayed spouses. But I couldn't dig out even a crumb of sympathy or longing or affection for this man. Just pity, relief even, for not ending up a greater part of his world. And proud for not having stooped to revenge. I'd attracted him into my life briefly, and it had purpose. For that I was grateful.

The chaos of kids exiting the field broke up further conversation with Melissa, but I'd heard all I needed. I had already relegated Graham to a storage box in the attic of my heart; now I could label it "the past."

Then, just days later—one day before my D-Day anniversary—my separation agreement with Robert was finalized. Crazy, the way the Universe works. I couldn't help but think it was winking in my direction. Sure, they're just "papers," and Robert and I had been emotionally and physically separated for a long time. But up until those papers were signed, I'd lived in constant fear of his threats: yanking spousal payments or demanding more custody of the kids. With the terms now clearly laid out, he could no longer threaten and bully me. I was now free to call the financial shots in my life, which was another huge step in my independence. My emotional energy could be channeled into my children and *me*; not the Passive Delaine who Robert thought I was, but the Empowered Delaine I had become.

Thus, my D-Day anniversary was not marked by nostalgia and loss, but by liberation and closure instead. Reaching that place hadn't been easy, but that Hellish journey was never meant to be my final destination: It was but a detour, a school of much-needed tough self-love, designed to bring me home—to myself.

By life throwing me flat on my face into an uncharted wilderness, I was tested to move beyond being a victim of circumstance to becoming the heroine of my own life and finding my way out the other side. I was stripped of my well-made excuses for remaining the deferential wife in an abusive marriage, and forced to look inward and outward for my *real* truth as a woman. My body became a catalyst for change, my sexual awakening a conduit for trust, liberation, and self-love. I was becoming whole again.

Hair and makeup done, I stood at my closet wearing my bright pink undergarments. *What should I wear on my date with Miss Hali?* My eyes suddenly stopped on the fuchsia pink wrap-shirt I'd worn on my first date with Hockey Player Cal. I smiled. Despite his small penis, how lucky was I to have met such a nice guy on my first date in ten years? Or any of the other men I'd dated this past year. In each of their ways—from the simple to the profound—they had all helped me to heal, learn, and grow.

Take my twelve "serial dates" from my first summer as a single mother. Though I only met each of them for one coffee date, *collectively* they helped boost my confidence and self-image as I adjusted to singlehood again.

Yummy Stranger followed. My spontaneous foray into young-man territory on a sunny afternoon wasn't just a step outside my boundaries, it was a leap: Body in the Red Zone, I boldly and aggressively took action, called the shots sexually, and satisfied my body's demands like a Woman Entitled. And in the aftermath, I didn't feel guilty or feel compelled to explain myself and justify my actions to Yummy Stranger; that alone felt empowering! My memories of that afternoon will always make me giggle; I never thought this stay-at-home could be so mischievous!

But the real shift in my life trajectory came when I met Shane, a.k.a., The Duke. Sure, he was extreme and unconventional, but his freaky mentorship helped me give *myself* permission to explore outside my comfort zone—sexually, psychologically, and emotionally. He helped me realize that there was a place in my sex life for my *brain*, not just my heart. That I could *choose* to either get swept away emotionally or embrace the experience as an opportunity for self-expression and physical pleasure alone. If it weren't for Shane, I probably would never have *allowed* myself to enjoy two different lovers in one weekend, surrender to an erotic night of passion in Vegas, or attempt to live out a hotel fantasy—all experiences that required me to shed oppressive mores that prevented me from exploring a deeper side of my sexual self—and ultimately, my deeper identity as a woman. Nor would I have tried to dominate my "service boys," Adonis-Boy Daniel and Minotaur Brent. These young men, in turn, not only warned me to my chameleon-like tendencies, they taught me about sex without attachment, sex for pleasure and play, and the importance of sex with good intentions.

Trust and self-awareness was further fostered by gentle hunky Football Coach Chad, whose G-spot "maneuvers" showed me just how far my body could go in expressing pleasure and abandon. *Who knew I was a squirter?!* Besides getting honorable mention in my personal history book, our soaking-hot nights reminded me that there's *always* more to learn: about my body, myself, and life.

Then, of course, there was zippity Dragonfly Lornce, whose playful joie de vivre came at a perfect time, when I was just on the cusp of feeling whole enough to simply be *me* and savor spontaneous moments with authentic joy in my heart instead of romantic idealism.

But no one had a greater impact on my efflorescence than Sir John the Dom, who helped me excavate the deeper me, allowing me to finally open up and trust again. He made me *feel* again—body, mind, and soul. And ultimately, through dominance and sexual submission, he helped me find and own more of my inner power, a dynamic I sense I'm not yet done exploring.

If you pull the lens far back on my life this past year and view the bigger picture, the entire journey was ultimately about submission: I had to "surrender" all of my old beliefs about who I was, and fully explore myself through my sexuality, sensuality, and "promiscuity" to begin rousing and claiming my personal power—not just as a woman, but as an *individual*. Not just Delaine the Stay-at-Home Mom or Delaine the Dutiful Wife, or even Delaine the Lover. Just *me*.

Through freeing my sexual energy, I also freed the other powerful energies of my sex chakra: creativity, enthusiasm, awe, passion, and pleasure. No, this wasn't just about sex or the physical, it was about full personal expression. I found myself experiencing a creative renaissance as I began channeling those energies into writing and blogging, and coaching other divorced women. I was living passionately: I was transmuting my sexual energy into *purpose*.

And it all started with my body. This beautiful, wise body of mine that I've spent a lifetime ignoring, suppressing, and physically trying to alter. My sexuality was the launch pad, the catalyst, that spurred growth in virtually every area of my life. It not only rescued me, it became my master spiritual teacher.

Thanks, Wild Woman, I thought, smiling, as I slid on a long black skirt and my red wrap-shirt. She'd guided me out of the wilderness, after all. But I believe she still had a thing or two to teach me.

HAVING ARRIVED AT the bar before Hali, I sat alone at my table, waiting for the server to return with my diet coke. *It's busy in here for a Wednesday*, I thought, as I leaned back in my chair and scanned the room. Immediately, I sensed being watched. Three thirty-something men had put their drinks down and were looking my way. Perhaps it was the energy I exuded, because I felt wonderful: fully alive, attractive, confident, and independent. I smiled and looked away. I was not at all interested in men tonight.

It feels good to be me, I thought, after the waitress dropped off my drink. *I'm sitting in a bar all by myself, a thirty-eight-year-old single mother of three. And it feels good to be in my skin.*

Suddenly, I glimpsed Hali at the bar's front entrance looking around. I stood and waved.

"Wow, hot stuff. You look great," she said, giving me a sly smile as she removed her coat. "Do you have a date after this or something?"

"No," I laughed. "But thanks! I just felt like fixing myself up a bit."

"So," she said, after ordering a glass of red wine. "How's dating life? Any interesting men or great lovers on the go?"

I leaned in and placed my glass on the table. "I really don't know where my dating life is heading these days, but I feel great. Grounded and happy. I'm not looking for anyone, you know? That said, it's been three months since I've had sex—"

"What!" she interrupted. "That's a shocker."

We both laughed.

"Honestly, Hali, men aside, the most important thing to me right now—beyond my kids—is establishing my career. I want to channel my passion and energy into something for *me* instead of a man. Don't get me wrong, I still want sex. And I want to date. But kids, my work, those are my priorities."

Hali smiled, and I could see in her eyes how happy and proud she was of me. Just as I was for her. She was still with Too-Good-to-Be-True Bobby, happy in the moment. And that's what counted. Sure, neither of was sure where our lives were headed, but the bottom line was that we'd made it through "Year One."

Spontaneously, I held up my glass. Without question, Hali raised hers up to mine, her blue eyes filled with warmth.

"To us," I said, "And our 'way better' life."

"To us . . ."

ACKNOWLEDGMENTS

As I PUT TOGETHER THIS acknowledgment's page, I find myself wiping away tears. It has been an exciting yet tumultuous road getting here, and I often wondered if this book wouldn't have been better off buried on a memory stick and forgotten.

Thus, it is with utmost gratitude that I share this book's publishing with my closest circle of girlfriends and my family. They have shared every bump, bruise, and triumph I've experienced along the journey, not just in writing this book but in dealing with the after tremors of my divorce. They know how much this book means to me, how it has changed me, added to me, and tested me in ways I'd never imagined. And celebrating its completion would be impossible—and meaningless—without them beside me.

Thus, to "Hali," "Tory," and "Tara," my beloved soul sisters, I send my heartfelt thanks for being my rocks, my mentors, and my closest confidantes. I'm so grateful for your wise counsel, nonjudgment, and infallible belief in me, not to mention all the mischief and belly laughs we've shared. Thanks as well for helping me find the courage to own the "nakedness" of this memoir. *ROAR!*

My thanks are further extended to all the gals in our girls group: "Selena," "Patti," "Shannon," Janet, Tara, and Shiloh, who each supported me in their own unique ways throughout this journey. Also, my gratitude goes to Miriam, my dear and old friend, and Tracy and Jason for being my surrogate family here in Calgary; the kids and I love you.

Of special note, my heartfelt thanks goes to my sister and mom. Since divorcing, my sister, Deborah, has helped me return to my center, time and time again. Moreover, she refused to let me do anything but shoot for the stars; thanks sis. And as for my mom, her support has been "extra" special. Despite the "raciness" of this book, she didn't flinch, question, or doubt me; rather, she just gave me constant thumbs up and said, "Keep going, I'm proud of you." Thanks as well to my dad, and my brothers, Chris and Keith, whose loving support from afar has been constant, even though they don't know the "details" of my book (*hehe*).

And to my dearest children, who are still too young to understand what this book is all about, I also send loving thanks. This book journey has stolen me away from family time; I've had to travel, work long hours, and sometimes I've been very distracted. But my utmost goal was to get me back to you—to being that loving and solid mom I've always tried so hard to be. I love you, my beautiful children; you are my heart.

I'd also like to express a special thanks to Brooke Warner, Eva Zimmerman, and the designers at Seal Press for their contributions in seeing this through to publication. And extra warm thanks goes out to my developmental editor, Merrik Bush-Pirkle, who helped me make this book mine, only more. Working with you has been an absolute joy.

Lastly, I want to say thanks to those of you who read this memoir. Please understand that I didn't write this memoir with an audience in mind or with the objective of selling it. So I feel completely honored that my story has ended up in your hands. I hope it has touched your heart or life in some way. Maybe even roused your Wild Woman. At the very least, I hope it made you stand a little taller.

XO —Delaine

ABOUT THE AUTHOR

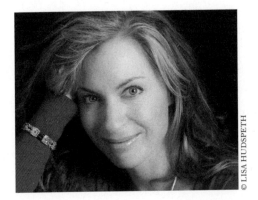

© LISA HUDSPETH

DELAINE MOORE is a Mars Venus Coach, speaker, journalist, and the fiery voice behind the popular blog, IAmDivorcedNot Dead.com, where she unabashedly gets down to the good, bad and "naughty" of life after divorce. Delaine writes for The Huffington Post, Your Tango, and First Wives World and has appeared on radio and television shows throughout North America. Delaine lives in Calgary, Alberta, with her three children. Follow her on Twitter @ Delaine_Moore.

SELECTED TITLES FROM SEAL PRESS

For more than thirty years, Seal Press has published
groundbreaking books. By women. For women.

Affection: An Erotic Memoir, by Krissy Kneen. $16.95, 978-1-58005-342-6.
A powerful, explicit, and sexy account of an extraordinarily sensual woman's
experiences with sex, from adolescence to adulthood, and an examination of how
her sense of self shapes and is shaped by those experiences.

Single Mom Seeking, by Rachel Sarah. $14.95, 978-1-58005-166-8. A single
mom shares her heartfelt and hilarious take on the challenges of balancing
motherhood with singlehood in her search for a good man.

Sex and Bacon: Why I Love Things That Are Very, Very Bad for Me, by
Sarah Katherine Lewis. $14.95, 978-1-58005-228-3. A sensual—and some-
times raunchy—book celebrating the intersection of sex and food.

Ask Me About My Divorce: Women Open Up About Moving On, edited
by Candace Walsh. $15.95, 978-1-58005-276-4. A spicy, bracing, riveting
anthology that proclaims: I got divorced, and it rocked my world!

Nice Girls, Naughty Sex: 20 Erotic Tales, edited by Jordan LaRousse and
Samantha Sade. $16.95, 978-1-58005-343-3. A fun, edgy anthology of erotic
literature compiled by the founders of the popular erotica website Oystersand-
Chocolate.com.

Open: Love, Sex, and Life in an Open Marriage, by Jenny Block. $16.95,
978-1-58005-275-7. Jenny Block recounts her personal experience with open
marriage and challenges our notions of what healthy marriage looks like.

FIND SEAL PRESS ONLINE
www.SealPress.com
www.Facebook.com/SealPress
Twitter: @SealPress